AROMA

MASSAGE CASE STUDIES

THE DEFINITIVE STUDY AID FOR
AROMATHERAPY STUDENTS & ENTHUSIASTS

<u>10 Real life case studies containing 40 individual treatments</u>

<u>FREE BONUS: 10 Aromatherapy Massage Client Consultation Forms</u>

By

EMMA LIVINGSTON

Copyright © 2016

INTRODUCTION

This book is a compilation of 10 case studies conducted by an Aromatherapy massage therapist. Each case study is a record of 4 massage treatments on each individual client so there are 40 treatments in total documented in this guide. This guide is very beneficial for any person training to become an aromatherapy therapist as it shows the process of dealing with clients from the initial consultation meeting to developing an aromatherapy treatment plan and adapting treatments to suit a clients needs.

Covered in detail are:

- Client Profile / Consultation form for each client- an overview of each client, their health and lifestyle.

- Reason for treatment: Main aims of the treatment -the client's requirements and main aims for each treatment.

- Treatment plan- therapists treatment plan with details on specific essential oil choices to suit the clients needs.

- Details of how the therapist conducted the treatment

- How the client felt during the treatment

- How the client felt after the treatment

- Homecare advice- advice for the client on using essential oils at home

- Reflective practice- therapists self reflection on how the treatment progressed and plans for the following treatments

- Conclusion- overall therapist self-reflection and learning outcomes after each 4-treatment case study.

Names have been changed to protect the privacy and identity of each individual client. This book is a guide to conducting treatments and in no way replaces conventional training. It is advised to conduct aromatherapy massage treatments only when training in the subject or qualified with appropriate insurance, as knowledge and expertise are required to perform treatments safely

TABLE OF CONTENTS

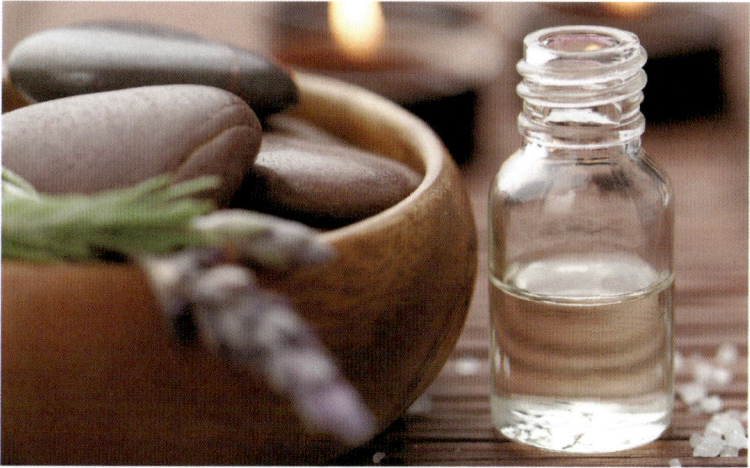

CASE STUDY 1

Client profile

Laura Ryan is 43 years old and has an active lifestyle, exercising regularly. She generally has good muscle tone but can get stiff and tense after exercise. She has a healthy diet and eats regular meals. She finds it easy to relax but she can be very stressed in work. She rates her stress level at work as 7 and her stress level at home as 1. She has no contraindications that require medical permission. She has Varicose Veins on her left leg, which is a contraindication that restricts the treatment to this area.

Reason for treatment: Main aims of the treatment

She requested a treatment that would boost her Immune system that would be invigorating and uplifting as she was feeling run down and tired lately. Also occasionally she will be coming for a treatment the same day she attends the gym so she wants a treatment that will help with tension/ stiffness. She finds when she becomes stressed in work she can feel a lot of tension build up in her back. I have chosen Almond Oil for the carrier oil. This oil is easily absorbed by the skin, balances the moisture of the body and is suitable for all skin types. I've chosen Bergamot, Black Pepper and Orange Sweet for this treatment. I did a patch test for black pepper at the initial consultation as the oil can cause skin sensitisation. Bergamot and Orange sweet are both phototoxic so I advised my client to avoid strong sunlight and sunbeds after the treatment.

Rationale for the choice of each essence:

Bergamot (Citrus Bergamia) - uplifting, immune system

Black Pepper (Piper Nigrum) stimulating, circulation, rubefacient.

Orange Sweet (Citrus Sinensis)- stress related conditions, refreshing.

Treatment plan:

<u>One</u> aromatherapy massage per week for four weeks; working on the legs, back, stomach, arms, face and head.

Oils / Botanical Name	Drops/ Mls	Uses
Bergamot / *Citrus Bergamia*	2 Drops	Anxiety, depression, immune system, uplifting nervous system.
Black Pepper / *Piper Nigrum*	3 Drops	Muscular aches/ pains, circulatory system, stimulating, coughs and colds
Orange Sweet / *Citrus Sinensis*	3 Drops	Digestion, nervous tension, stress related conditions, refreshing
Sweet Almond / *Prunus Commmunis*	25 mls	Protective, nourishing, vitamins- A, B1, B2, B6, E

TREATMENT 1
Details of how the therapist conducted the treatment

My client said she had no reaction to the patch test I did for black pepper so I went ahead to use it for the treatment. First I let my client smell the blend I used for the oils and she liked the smell, if a client dislikes particular smells they are unlikely to relax during the treatment or enjoy it. She arrived for the treatment saying she had stiff calf muscles and tension in her shoulders and upper arms. She was in the gym the previous day and felt she had probably over exerted. I performed a full body massage with emphasis on the specific areas of tension. I was only able to break down the adhesions with friction movements on her right leg. My client has Varicose Veins on her lower left leg, which is a restrictive contraindication so I avoided her lower leg completely. I did extra Petrissage movements (finger rolling, thumb rolling, wringing and frictions) on her trapezius and rhomboid muscles and around her scapulae bones, as this is where she had a lot of tension and adhesions. This combined with the rubefacient affects of Black Pepper oil helped to break down lactic acid and reduce muscular aches and pains.

This happens by the blood being warmed by the oil, circulation improves so there is quicker delivery of oxygen and nutrients and a faster removal of CO_2 and waste. Bergamot and Orange Sweet have similar properties both are used for strengthening and protecting the immune system and citrus oils help a client feel uplifted and are stress reducing. These oils affect how the body works by changing impulses and messages sent around the body. The relaxing/distressing properties of the oils can help to relieve symptoms of stress on the body. When I finished the treatment I helped my client off the massage table and gave her a glass of water to drink.

How the Client felt during the treatment

My client was very chatty at the start of the treatment but relaxed after a few minutes and was quite for the remainder of the treatment. She didn't like lying face down on the massage table as she felt congested so I got her to lie with her face to one side.

How the client felt after the treatment

Her mood definitely lifted after the massage and she said she really liked the fruity smell off the oils so I will be using the same combination for next treatment. She said in the initial consultation that she has good circulation but she mentioned during the massage that she has cold hands and feet. Black Pepper used in this treatment is stimulating and helps with circulation problems. She said she felt relaxed but also quite alert and didn't feel tired after the treatment. She mentioned she didn't like having her head massaged and requested I leave that out in future.

Homecare advice

I gave my client a glass of water to drink while I went through the homecare advice with her. I advised her to drink more water and try to cut down on caffeine and alcohol. She rated her stress level in work as a 7, which is quite high. I asked her to look for different aspects in work that might be causing a high stress level such as workload, doing overtime, delegating to colleagues and is she taking regular breaks during the way. I think if she becomes more aware of what is causing the most stress she is in a better position to make changes. I advised her to take the time to do warm up, cool down exercises in the gym to keep supple after a workout. I discussed possible reactions; heightened emotions, thirst, fatigue, skin breakouts. I explained these would pass within 24 hours and are normal reactions to treatments. I gave her a sheet with the names of the oils I have used in the treatment and their benefits. I suggested she could use 3 drops of Bergamot or Orange Sweet in the bath if she is stressed after work to lift her spirits.

Reflective practice

The music stopped during the treatment I will remember next time to keep it on repeat. I was restricted in moving around the bed in the room so I need to practice in a room with more space. I had the height of the bed too low so my posture wasn't good throughout the treatment.

TREATMENT 2

Any changes to consultation

There are no changes to the consultation apart from my client requesting we leave out the head massage.

Reactions to last treatment

She felt stressed before the last treatment but she said she was more relaxed and calmer after the treatment. She added Bergamot drops to her bath during the week, which she said helped her relax and unwind after work. She also felt warm and flushed for a few hours after the massage, which I feel, was a reaction to the Black Pepper. She felt that after the treatment and the next day her upper back and shoulders felt looser and not as tense.

Details of the treatment

My client arrived after attending the gym. She seemed fairly agitated and said she had been rushing to make our appointment. I asked her to take a few deep breaths to help her relax. I started the massage routine with extra Effleurage movements to soothe and relax her. I decided to use the same oils again in this treatment.

Orange sweet and Bergamot oils have similar properties both are stress reducing and are uplifting and refreshing. When I was doing the facial massage she could fully inhale the oils. Smell is the fastest way for essential oils to penetrate the body. The molecules in the oils send messages to the brain and from the lungs they pass to the bloodstream. Depending on the interpretation of the oil the brain will send messages to parts of the body to create a response. In this instance the responses to these oils would be deeper breathing, mind clearing, positive feelings and muscles relaxing. This was evident with my client as at the start her breathing was rapid and she felt very tense and by the end of the massage this had reduced noticeably.

She didn't have any adhesions or appear to be tender in her back or calf muscles like she had been last week but she said she had been doing stretches after the gym and regularly going to the sauna after a workout which seemed to help. Also she did some hot compresses for her back when she felt tense. She made an appointment for the following week.

How the client felt during the treatment

She was quite straight away and seemed to relax very quickly. She fell asleep during the massage and I had to wake her to turn her over on the table even though the blend is supposed to be Stimulate and Uplifting. But she said she hadn't slept well during the week so this could be a contributing factor.

How the client felt after the treatment

Before the treatment she appeared slightly agitated she was talking very fast and said she had been in low spirits for two days before this treatment due to personal problems. The massage calmed her right down and she was in very good spirits after the massage.

Homecare advice

My client felt thirsty after the treatment so I gave her water to drink. I gave her a sheet outlining general homecare advice and possible reactions. When she is stressed she gets headaches and also tension in her upper back. I told her not to shower for 24 hours after the treatment to get the full benefit of the oils. I gave her advice on how to make Compresses; Hot compresses for muscle aches and pains with one drop of black pepper and also how to make a cold compress for which is good for headaches with a drop of Marjoram. Marjoram is good for headaches, stress and it is also relaxing.

Reflective practice

I had quite a stressful day and I felt as a result this affected the massage. My client didn't mention that there was any difference but I felt tenser and my posture wasn't good throughout. I need to be more aware of this and try to find ways to reduce my stress level as I ended up feeling very tired afterwards and my back was very sore.

TREATMENT 3

Any changes to consultation

There are no changes to the initial consultation.

Reactions to last treatment

She felt very hot and flushed again after the last treatment and decided to have a shower soon afterwards to cool down, which would have compromised the benefits of the oils. She said she felt very alert after the massage, didn't sleep well and had a headache the next day after the treatment. This can sometimes be a normal reaction to massage that will pass.

I decided to change Black pepper from the previous treatments to Lavindin. Black pepper is a strong rubefacient oil and my client didn't like how flushed she felt after the massage so I feel it would be better to try another oil. I choose Lavandin as it is beneficial for her muscular system and would help with headaches and stress. Lavindin also has the properties of lavender without being a strong sedative so it is safer to use during the day. There are no known safety factors with the oil.

Oils/ Botanical Name	Drops/ Mls	Uses
Bergamot *Citrus Bergamia*	3 Drops	Anxiety, depression, immune system, uplifting nervous system.
Lavindin *Lavandula x intermedia*	2 Drops	Muscular system, circulatory system, headaches, analgesic
Orange Sweet *Citrus Sinensis*	3 Drops	Digestion, nervous tension, stress related conditions, refreshing
Sweet Almond *Prunus Commmunis*	25 mls	Protective, nourishing, vitamins- A, B1, B2, B6, E

Details of the treatment

My client arrived for an evening appointment in good form. She said that she hadn't been to the gym this week as she had a fairly stressful week at work, and was very tired most days. She mentioned her neck was very stiff and she hadn't good posture this week. I explained to her I would be changing Black pepper to Lavandin and to notice if she would have any reactions to it over the next week. I preformed a Full body massage leaving out the scalp massage as she doesn't like it. I checked my pressure of the movements with the client throughout. The Splenius Capitas, rhomboids and trapezius muscles were very tense in comparison to the previous weeks. I did extra petrissage movements over theses muscles to improve the circulation, breakdown fibrous build up and eliminate lactic acid from tension. Lavandin used in this treatment is an analgesic and rubefacient so it is good for muscle pains and stiffness. The oil once absorbed into the bloodstream from the skin has a similar affect as the petrissage massage movements- the blood is warmed by the oil, it moves faster so oxygen /nutrients are brought to stiff muscles and waste in the muscles is removed faster. She seemed to have poor circulation at her Latissimus Dorsi and external oblique's so I applied more pressure to work the tissues adequately and warm the area. When I had finished the massage I helped my client off the massage table and gave her a glass of water to drink.

How the client felt during the treatment

She had adhesions in the splenius capitis and rhomboid muscles she said she had a lot of stiffness in her neck this week and found it hard to rotate her neck. I noticed her lower back (Latissimus Dorsi muscles and side of external oblique's) were a much colder area than the rest of her body which would suggest poor circulation there. She talked a lot for the first 10 minutes but gradually stopped and relaxed. She seemed to be hunching when lying face down but after the back massage she no longer seemed as tense.

How the client felt after the treatment

She said she especially liked the work I did around her neck from the trapezius muscles to her occipital bones. She felt she had a lot of tension in her forehead which she felt had eased after the massage. I was a bit conscious that I didn't want her to be too tired after the massage as it was early evening and she would be driving home afterwards. But she didn't appear tired at all after the massage just lot calmer.

Homecare advice

I gave my client a sheet outlining general reactions and homecare advice. I noticed her skin was very dry and parched and soaked up the oil very quickly. She does admit that she generally doesn't drink anything bar coffee, soft drinks and alcohol. These can dehydrate her body and the affects are evident on her skin. I asked her to consider having a glass of water when she is also having another drink. I advised her again about trying out hot and cold compresses as she will find them beneficial between treatments.

Reflective practice

I had tension and pain in the middle of my back while I did the massage this has happened quite often but it is something I am becoming more aware of the more treatments I do. I have also found my breathing isn't regular. I am going to try yoga and breathing exercises as I need to become more relaxed while doing a treatment and also need to strengthen the muscles in my upper back and arms. I realised towards the end of the routine that I had forgot to sanitise my client's hands. Apart from that I think the massage went well and my client was happy to make another appointment for the following week

TREATMENT 4

Any changes to consultation

There are no changes to the consultation from last week. My client is happy enough to go ahead with the treatment with the same massage oils as the previous week.

Reactions to last treatment

She said she felt good and her mood had lifted after the last massage and she didn't feel tired that evening after the massage. She said she felt this way for most of the week. She had felt tension across her forehead before the last massage but this had lifted afterwards. She said her back muscles were much looser and less tense after the massage but later in the week she started to feel stiff again.

Details of the treatment

My client arrived for the massage in good spirits and was very chatty at the start. She said she had been dancing for two nights in a row and said she felt stiff all over and in some pain, but not as much pain as the previous week. I performed a full body massage leaving out the scalp as requested. I started with extra effleurage movements to help her relax for the treatment.

Boosting circulation with petrissage movements helped to relieve stiffness in her muscles by removing toxins and delivering oxygen and nutrients to the muscles quicker. I used Lavandin again for this treatment. This oil is an antispasmodic so it prevents and relieves spasms which can occur in tired overworked muscles. Bergamot and lavandin have analgesic properties so they will help to relieve muscular pain. I noticed that it wasn't as tender in the splenius capitis, trapezius and rhomboid muscles this week and I was able to apply more pressure with the movements to the area. She has still being using hot compresses for her upper back muscles with a few drops of Lavandin on the compress. When I finished the massage I helped my client off the massage table.

How the client felt during the treatment

She was very chatty during the treatment but started to quieten down when I did the back massage. She said she had a stiff back and legs- the muscles were tight in these areas but I was able to work the tension out quite easily.

How the client felt after the treatment

She said she didn't feel tense after the massage. She was calmer and more relaxed than she had been at the start of the massage.

Homecare advice

Her skin wasn't as dry this week as she has started using moisturising cream. She started drinking more water than she has previously which will help to rehydrate her skin. As this was the last treatment I went through the last four treatments with her explaining to her what I had noticed over the treatments such as where she has experienced tension in her body and her stress levels and ways of helping to relieve the symptoms- Hot and Cold compresses using essential oils and putting essential oils into the bath. I gave her a list of suitable oils for stress, tension, muscular aches/pains that will be beneficial for her to use. Also I talked to her about taking regular breaks in work and doing stretches for her neck and upper back to keep it supple and help her relax. I had some of the oil left over from this last treatment which I gave to her in a bottle to use, I explained she could place the oil into a burner to inhale and get the benefits of the oils.

Reflective practice

I made a conscious effort to relax as much as possible during the massage and keep my arms loose while I worked. I found it helped a lot and I didn't experience any pain or tension as a result. I found I wasn't as tired and I feel my routine has improved as a result. I feel I rushed the massage I was finished about ten minutes sooner than I expected. I was conscious of the fact I was doing another massage straight after this one so that's why I felt rushed. In future I think I need to allow at least 30 mins between finishing one treatment and starting another.

OVERALL CONCLUSION

T1: My client arrived for the first treatment stiff and tense all over. After the massage treatment she felt her mood had lifted and she felt relaxed and alert.

T2: Before the massage my client felt agitated, she relaxed quickly and was very calm and was in good spirits afterwards. She had taken on some of my homecare advice for hot compresses and stretching exercises in the gym which had helped her overall tension/ stiffness.

T3: I changed Black pepper to Lavandin. She has a stiff neck and said she had a stressful week. After the massage tension in her forehead had eased and she seemed calmer. She hadn't done any of my suggestions for homecare advice from the previous week.

T4: My client was experiencing overall stiffness when she arrived, after the treatment she didn't feel tense and was calmer and relaxed. As for homecare advice I gave her suggestions on using aromatherapy oils to help with stress relief and muscular tension. She has taken on board my advice some weeks but I think the most important thing for her is to become more aware of how she feels physically and mentally and try to make small changes every week to help herself.

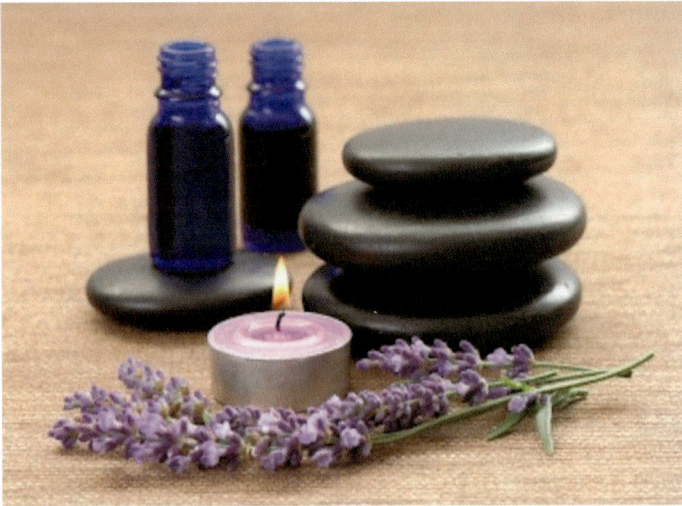

CASE STUDY 2:

CLIENT PROFILE

Jenny Neary is in her late Thirties and has just had her first baby five months ago. She lives with her husband and is stepmother to his daughter. She is planning to stay at home and look after her baby but she may be returning to work part time shortly. She doesn't have a babysitter generally and looks after her baby herself during the week and occasionally gets a break when her husband isn't working at the weekends. Her sleeping pattern is unsettled as her baby wakes often at night and when she gets a particularly bad night's sleep she gets headaches the following day .

She isn't stressed in general but she does feel that the lack of sleep leaves her feeling agitated occasionally and that she needs some time in her life where she can relax and unwind. She has gained a small amount of weight since having her baby and she rarely gets a chance to exercise since she had her baby. She says she generally doesn't have any pain or stiffness in her muscles apart from her arms and the cervical area of her neck occasionally.

Reason for treatment: main aims of the treatment

She has a poor sleep pattern and gets headaches when she sleeps particularly badly so helping with this is a main aim for the treatments.

Rationale for the choice of each essence:

Mandarin- Insomnia

Marjoram- Headaches helps Insomnia

Peppermint- Headaches, Cephalic

I checked the safety factors of these Oils with my Client and she didn't have any contraindications to the oils. Peppermint should not be used when a Client is taking homeopathic remedies. Marjoram cannot be used if a client is pregnant as it brings on menstruation. Mandarin is phototoxic so shouldn't be used before exposure to sunlight.

Treatment plan:

A full body massage including the face over 4 weeks. Massage movements that will be used are Effleurage, Petrissage and Frictions.

Oils / Botanical Name	Drops/ Mls	Uses
Mandarin _Citrus reticulata_	3 Drops	Anxiety, Insomnia, stomach ailments, uplifting, refreshing, stretch marks, oedema, digestive
Marjoram _Origanum marjorana_	3 Drops	Muscular aches/pains, headaches, circulation, relaxant, helps insomnia, stress
Peppermint _Mentha piperita_	2 Drops	Indigestion, flatulence, headaches, cooling/refreshing, Cephalic, nervous system, immune system
Sweet Almond _Prunus Commmunis_	25 mls	Protective, nourishing, vitamins- A,B1,B2, B6, E

TREATMENT 1
Details of how the therapist conducted the treatment

I performed the massage in my clients own home. It was more convenient for my client as she only had a babysitter for an hour. I prepared the massage table in her spare room making sure I had enough towels and the room was warm. I aimed to perform a full body massage before I started I washed my hands and sanitised my client's feet. I helped my client onto the massage table (protecting her modesty). I covered all body parts and only removed certain towels when I was massaging a particular area. I placed supports under her head, ankles and knees when needed. I let my client smell the blend before I started the massage and she liked it so I proceeded to use the oils.

The main emphasis for the aromatherapy treatment is to introduce my client to oils that will help her sleep better and also help reduce headaches. I have used three oils here that are specifically for poor sleeping and headaches- Mandarin, Marjoram and Peppermint. I choose Mandarin for its refreshing fruity aroma inhaling this oil helps to lift anxiety and its sedative relaxing properties helps with sleep patterns.

Marjoram and Mandarin oils act as a depressant for the central nervous system- they decrease nerve impulses through the spine, brain and associated organs so as a result the person becomes more relaxed less nervous, making it easier to fall asleep and remain asleep.

My client was very stiff in the Trapezius, Deltoid and Rhomboid muscles so I did a lot of Petrissage and Frictions to break down adhesions and reduce stiffness in these areas. I have used Marjoram to help with my clients sleeping pattern but it is also beneficial for muscular aches and pains. The oil absorbs into the skin and dilates the tiny capillaries close to the skins surface creating a feeling of local warmth. The increase of local circulation helps to carry away the toxic wastes left in the muscles and thus reducing stiffness and pain.

How the client felt during the treatment

My client was fairly uneasy; her baby was being minded down stairs and she could hear her occasionally. She was listening out to make sure her baby wasn't crying downstairs so this distracted her away from the massage. She had experienced massages before so she wasn't apprehensive about the treatment and was very interested in the different techniques that I used.

How the client felt after the treatment.

She said she felt much more relaxed and calmer after the treatment as she was fairly tense beforehand.

Homecare advice

After I was finished the massage I helped my client to get down off the massage table onto couch roll. Once she was dressed I talked to her about aftercare, possible reactions and homecare advice. I gave her a glass of water to flush out any accumulating toxins. I suggested to her to try and have the massage when there isn't likely to be any disruptions as it will help her relax more and she will get more benefit from the massage. She doesn't often get a break from looking after her baby so a weekly massage will help her release tension and stress that she might accumulate. I have suggested to my client to get an oil burner in her bedroom and inhale the oils for an hour before going to bed to help her sleep and also to help with headaches.

The oils I advised her for the burner are peppermint and mandarin which are the two oils I used in the treatment. I gave her the oil I had left over from the treatment to use first in the oil burner and I asked her to let me know if the blend helps with her sleep pattern and headaches. I asked her to write down over the next few weeks when she gets headaches such as after eating certain foods, stressful incidences, lack of sleep etc. and also her routine for going to sleep-what can be can trigger her sleep pattern.

Reflective practice

My client said she was pleased with the massage as she explained she doesn't get much of a break to relax after having her baby. My client talked throughout the massage so next time I will play relaxing music so hopefully she can unwind more and might not be inclined to talk throughout as I found it hard to concentrate on the moves while she made conversation.

TREATMENT 2

Any changes to consultation

There is only one change to the initial consultation-
my client said she had period pain this week and
requested I left out the abdomen massage.

Reactions to last treatment

She said she had positive reactions to the last
treatment. She slept well the night after the massage.
She had put the oils I had given her in the oil burner
and had inhaled them for a few nights. She said she
felt calmer and as a result didn't have any headaches
during the week. So I will use the same oils for this
treatment.

Details of the treatment

I prepared the massage table and side table as
before. I needed to add an extra heater to the room,
as it was a bit cold. I did a full body massage in an
hour. My client had no obvious tension so I conducted
the full body massage without extra emphasis on any
particular area.

My client had her period and she felt quite tender so she felt it was best not to do the abdomen massage on this occasion. I gave her advice on making a hot compress for period cramps. Marjoram and Mandarin oils that I have used for this treatment help with period pain; Mandarin specifically for PMT and Marjoram is an analgesic so it relieves pain. The oils are absorbed into the blood steam via the skin and the chemical constituents of the oil interact with the body's chemistry creating the desired effect.

I spent longer doing the face and décolletage massage. She said she was starting to get a tension headache before I started the massage. The essential oil molecules are inhaled and travel through the nasal passage to a receptor neuron that transport to the limbic part of the brain. Peppermint that I have used has analgesic and cephalic properties. These molecules would be picked up by the hypothalamus, which would transmit messages to the rest of the brain and body to relieve pain, relax, calm and settle the mind. In turn this would relieve the tension headache build up.

When I had finished the massage I helped my client off the massage table and gave her a glass of water to drink.

How the client felt during the treatment

Her breathing was fairly rapid at the start of the massage but she started to breath slower during the massage. She said had period pain, which was causing her discomfort. She requested I didn't do the abdomen massage on this occasion and this is a contraindication for not doing the massage in this area.

How the client felt after the treatment

After the massage she was relaxed and seemed to be in good spirits. She said she enjoyed the face massage the most. She said that before the face massage she was starting to get a headache and she felt that the massage I did on her forehead especially helped to alleviate this as the tension that was starting to build up started to relieve and her mind had cleared. The massage movements I did on her forehead were palmer kneading and pressure points on the medial and lateral frontal bone.

Homecare advice

Since she had slept well this week and hadn't had any headaches so she hadn't noticed anything that triggered them. She had taken on board my suggestion about using an oil burner in her room at night, she said she felt calmer and more relaxed and as a result she didn't experience headaches during the week or she felt she slept better this week.

She said she felt light headed after the massage so I asked her not to take on anything too strenuous for the rest of the day and not to drive till she felt that feeling had passed. She was concerned that she had a breakout of spots on her back after the last massage, I explained to her that can be reaction after the massage as the skin has been stimulated increasing sebum production but her skin's overall texture and tone would start to improve after a few massages. She went for a walk twice this week with her baby and she hopes to go more this week but she is pleased that she has started back exercising. I gave her advice on making compresses this week. She said she experienced quite sever period pains and I suggested a hot compress for her abdomen with one drop of Rose cabbage, rose damask or marjoram as they can help relieve uterine problems and PMT.

Reflective practice

I played relaxing music, which did help my client to relax, she was quite this week so I was able to concentrate more and I feel I did a better massage this week. I didn't do the abdomen massage this week as my client had period pain. I think it is important to ask clients how they feel before starting the massage, as there can sometimes be contraindications since the last massage that can restrict the treatment and it is important that the client isn't put under any unnecessary discomfort during the massage.

Any changes to consultation

There are no changes to initial consultation.

Reactions to last treatment

My client said she slept well the night of the massage but during the week she hadn't and also she had a headache during the week. She had put peppermint alone in the oil burner before going to sleep; it does help with mental fatigue and headaches but it can also refreshes the mind and wakes a person up, so I have advised her not to use this at night in future but use the Mandarin and Marjoram instead as they specifically help with Sleep problems. Also this appointment is in the evening this time so I am going to change peppermint to Eucalyptus oil. My client also said her muscles were stiff and sore this week so I have chosen this oil for headaches and muscular aches and pains. Mandarin is phototoxic so I advised my client to avoid strong sunlight and sunbeds. I checked to make sure my client wasn't taking homeopathic remedies as it is a safety factor to Eucalyptus and marjoram needs to be avoided during pregnancy. None of these issues were relevant to my client so I used them.

Oils Botanical Name	Drops/ Mls	Uses
Mandarin *Citrus reticulata*	3 Drops	Anxiety, Insomnia, stomach ailments, uplifting, refreshing, stretch marks, oedema, digestive
Marjoram *Origanum marjorana*	3 Drops	Muscular aches/pains, headaches, circulation, relaxant, helps insomnia, stress
Eucalyptus *Eucalyptus dives*	2 Drops	Muscular aches pains, Headaches, Migraines , Respiratory system Immune system and the Skin
Sweet Almond *Prunus Commmunis*	25 mls	Protective, nourishing, vitamins-A,B1,B2, B6, E

Details of the treatment

I did the massage in the early evening so I had soft lighting in the room. I prepared the massage table and side table as before and I played relaxing music. I did a full body massage including the abdomen (this was left out last week). I checked my pressure doing the massage movements throughout to make sure it was within my client's tolerance. I changed Peppermint to Eucalyptus in this treatment. I checked to make sure my client wasn't taking any homeopathic remedies, as this oil isn't suitable to use with any. My client liked the smell of the blend of oils. It is important to let the client smell the blend of oils because if they like the smell of the oils this will help the client to relax and provoke a positive response. Eucalyptus is an analgesic so it helps relieve headaches. When the oil is inhaled the molecules of the oil cause a response in an overactive nervous system. When pain is felt the oil slows down the reaction of pain receptors in the brain and this in turn relieves the pain.

She had tension and stiffness in her hamstrings and calf muscles. I started the massage on the back of her thighs with Effleurage. This move combined with the rubefacient properties of Eucalyptus warms the skin and increases blood and lymph flow around the body. Oxygen is increased in the blood helps to remove lactic acid build up and waste in muscles. I did palmer kneading, picking up and wringing (petrissage movements) after Effleurage. These movements are relaxing and help to break down adhesions and reduce stiffness. When I was finished the massage I helped my client off the bed to stand on couch roll.

How the client felt during the treatment

She appeared to be very tired at the start of the massage and she was a bit grumpy also she said she wasn't feeling the best as she hadn't slept well. She said her legs were sore and stiff. She has started using her exercise bike at home but she feels she might have done too much too soon as her legs are stiff and sore especially her Gastrocnemius and Hamstring muscles.

How the client felt after the treatment

She was quite during the massage and she said she felt very relaxed afterwards. Her mood had lifted and she seemed happier. She said she felt calm and her muscles didn't feel as stiff afterwards.

Homecare advice

For the rest of the day I told my client to drink plenty of water and eat light easily digestible foods. She noticed that she had been going to bed at different times during the week and had eaten late on two occasions. She hasn't yet got her baby into a set routine so her baby can be unsettled at night. Lack of routine and trying to digest food late at night can affect sleeping patterns greatly and can lead to fatigue, lack of concentration and tension headaches. I talked to her about starting to get a set routine of going to bed at a similar time, waking at a certain time and trying to eat before 7pm will help with her sleep pattern. The skin breakout she had last week had improved. She has increased her water intake this week. She has started to increase her exercise levels, she is using her exercise bike at home, along with continuing to go for walks and she is feeling stiff as a result I suggested she could take a warm bath in the evenings to relax her muscles before bed and it would also help relax her for sleep.

I suggested she adds up to 6 drops of Lavender to an unscented shower gel to put into the bath. Lavender has relaxing, sedative properties and will help relieve headaches and help her to sleep better. Also it helps with easing muscular aches and pains. I talked to her about the importance of warm up and cool down exercises before and after exercise as she begins to improve her fitness levels.

Reflective practice

She didn't talk during the massage, which helped me to concentrate more on the routine. I broke the routine to get extra oil for her skin and it is important not to break contact with the client because as soon as the hands are removed the body registers that is the end of the massage and begin to change gear.

TREATMENT 4

Any changes to consultation

The only change to the consultation is she sprained her ankle during the week this is a restrictive contraindication.

Reactions to last treatment

She said she slept well the night of the massage. The next day she had a migraine but she did a cold compress for her forehead and it eased off. She was pleased that she could use the essential oils to help relieve it without taking pain killer medication. Her sleeping pattern wasn't good later in the week as her baby had been very unsettled and sick and was waking up more at night.

Details of the treatment

I prepared the massage table and side table as before. I did the massage again in my client's home. I added an extra heater to the room, as it was cold.

My client told me before the massage that she had sprained her ankle during the week since the last massage apart from that I did a full body massage. An ankle sprain is a contraindication that restricts treatment so I avoided doing a massage near her ankle.

I made a hot compress for her ankle with one drop of marjoram oil on it. Marjoram can be used specifically for sprains due to its analgesic and warming properties. I changed the compress a few times when I was doing the massage to keep her ankle warm. I checked throughout with my client to make sure I was applying the right amount of pressure. She had adhesions and tension in her upper back around the rhomboids/ trapezius which I worked out with frictions and petrissage. These movements manipulate and tone muscle break down lactic acid and improve blood and lymph flow. After the massage I cleaned off any excess oil on her feet then I helped my client off the bed onto couch roll and gave her water to drink.

How the client felt during the treatment

My client's baby had been unsettled during the week so my client felt stressed and hadn't slept much. As a result she was quite tense and didn't relax fully till near the end of the massage when she fell asleep. She sprained her ankle so this was causing her pain, so I avoided massaging this area. She wasn't conscious that she had tension in her upper back muscles till I worked over the rhomboids and trapezius with petrissage and friction movements, which became painful to touch so I reduced my pressure there. She hadn't got to do much exercise this week since she sprained her ankle so her calf and thigh muscles weren't tense.

How the client felt after the treatment

She fell asleep during the massage as she was very tired and also there are sedative properties in the oils which helped to relax her. She said she enjoyed this massage the most as this massage has been her only time since last week to relax.

Homecare advice

I gave her advice on using an essential oil in a safe way to help her baby relax and sleep better. For a baby under 3 years of age – 10 drops in a 100mls of distilled water can be sprayed around the babies room as a mist and onto linen, I have suggested Lavender oil as it is neither toxic or irritating, relaxes breathing and it's a relaxing sedative suitable for babies. She was pleased with the suggestion and said she will try it out. I suggested a few drops of lavender oil on my client's pillow will also help her to sleep and continuing to work on getting a set routine that I suggested last week. She sprained her ankle this week so she didn't get to do any exercise but I advised her not to put too much pressure on that foot and only start exercising when her doctor recommends it. I talked to her about applying a hot compress on her ankle to help with the healing process.

Also soaking her foot in a bowl of warm water for 20minutes every night with two drops of Marjoram mixed with an unscented liquid soap will help ease the sprain. I advised her to relax for the rest of the evening and not do anything too strenuous if possible as she was very tired after her week. She said she is pleased with having regular massages as it is her only time at the moment to unwind without any distractions.

Reflective practice

I was pleased with how the massage went overall. My client has long hair which I forgot to tie up before I started the massage so it was a bit awkward trying to do that during the massage so I will remember this for next time.

Overall conclusion

T1: She was tense during the massage but felt more relaxed afterwards.

T2: She took on board my homecare advice and had a positive response to the oils. She had period pain and a headache and I gave her suggestions for using the oils for pain relief.

T3: I changed Peppermint to Eucalyptus, as Peppermint isn't suitable for an evening appointment. She hadn't slept well during the week and was very tired and grumpy at the start of the massage, afterwards her mood had lifted and she felt relaxed. I gave her advice on doing a daily routine to help her sleep better and suggestions for using the oils.

T4: She didn't sleep well during the week due to her baby being unsettled but she fell asleep during the massage. She sprained her ankle during the week so I did a hot compress to help with the swelling and pain. I gave her advice on using Lavender oil to help her baby relax and sleep better. My client was willing to take on board my homecare advice and she had positive responses to the advice and also to each massage treatment.

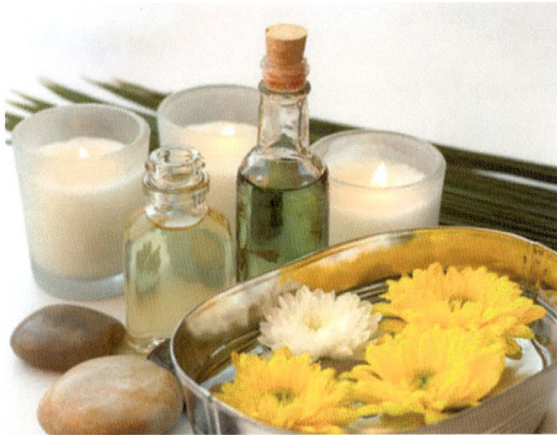

CASE STUDY 3:

CLIENT PROFILE

Pauline Quine has come to me for aromatherapy massage treatments as she suffers from muscular aches and pains in her back. She is also very stressed in work and has poor posture which has contributed to the pain. She finds it hard to fully relax and doesn't sleep very well during her working week. She finds at the weekends when she isn't in work she sleeps very well and relaxes much easier. She works as a credit controller and feels very dissatisfied and overworked at times in her job. She also spends long hours at her desk everyday and currently doesn't do any exercise so she often feels stiff and tense.

Reason for treatment: Main aims of the treatment

She requested a Treatment that would help her relax and also help reduce her stress levels. She also has muscular pain regularly in her back and wants treatments that will help alleviate this. I have chosen Almond Oil for the carrier oil. This oil is easily absorbed by the skin, balances the moisture of the body and is suitable for all skin types for this treatment. For the aromatherapy oils I have chosen Eucalyptus, Marjoram and Neroli. Eucalyptus is not compatible with homeopathic treatments. Marjoram needs to be avoided during pregnancy and Neroli has no known safety factors, I checked these with my client before I proceeded with the treatment.

Rationale for the choice of each essence:

Eucalyptus (eucalyptus smithii) - Muscular System, Aches and pains, Stress

Marjoram (Origanum marjorana) - Muscular aches and pains, relaxant, stress relief

Neroli (Citrus Aurantium) – Stress relief, insomnia, relaxing

Treatment Plan:

One aromatherapy massage per week for four weeks; working on the legs, back, stomach, arms, face and head

Oils / Botanical Name	Drops/ Mls	Uses
Eucalyptus *eucalyptus smithii*	3 Drops	Muscular system, aches/pains, respiratory system, stress, immune system
Marjoram *Origanum marjorana*	2 Drops	Headaches, circulation, relaxant, helps insomnia, stress, Muscular aches/pains
Neroli *Citrus Aurantium*	3 Drops	Stress relief, anxiety, insomnia, nervous system, relaxant, emotional upsets.
Sweet Almond *Prunus Commmunis*	25 mls	Protective, nourishing, vitamins- A, B1, B2, B6, E

TREATMENT 1
Details of how the therapist conducted the treatment

I covered my client with the appropriate towels and sanitised her hands and feet. I performed a full body massage apart from the stomach massage as she requested I left it out of the treatment. The movements I used were Effleurage and Petrissage which are slower movements that help the client relax and unwind. The main emphasis of an aromatherapy massage is to use the oils to create desired effects. In this massage the emphasis was on helping to reduce muscular pain and bring down her stress levels. Eucalyptus, marjoram, and Neroli all have stress reduction properties. Eucalyptus and Marjoram also are beneficial for muscular aches and pains. My client smelled the blend first and she really liked it. This response to smelling the oil will help her relax as it creates a positive association. These essential oils can affect how the body works by changing the chemical messages and impulses sent around her body relieving her stress by slowing her heart rate and breathing rate. The more she inhaled the oils she started to reduce her breathing rate and she started to get very sleepy.

The Rubefacient effects of Eucalyptus and Marjoram brought warmth and redness to her skin as a result blood vessels dilate. More oxygen and nutrients are then brought to the area and removing waste which is especially beneficial for reducing muscular aches and pains in her back. I worked her back for much longer with extra petrissage movements especially frictions around her scapulae as she had lots of adhesions. Petrissage movements break down adhesions and manipulate and tone muscles. This combined with the oils produced erythema- increasing blood and lymph flow around her body .By the end of the treatment my client was tired so I gave her a few minutes on her own to become more alert and bring her awareness back to her surroundings.

How the client felt during the treatment

She chatted a lot to start with but started to relax and quieten down after about ten minutes. She was very tender in her trapezius, splenius capitis, external obliques and latissimus dorsi muscles in her back. She asked me to reduce my pressure when I was working around the trapezius as she was in pain. I increased my petrissage movements there but reduced down the pressure to what she could handle. She also had a cold and was very congested as a result so she found it hard to breathe when she was lying face down on the table.

How the client felt after the treatment

After the treatment she said she felt calmer and more relaxed. She said she still felt stiff around her shoulders and lower back but she wasn't in as much pain as she had been before the treatment. She was still as congested as she was before the massage even though I had used Eucalyptus oil which is often used for its decongestant properties. She was very sleepy after the massage and took a few minutes to become more alert.

Homecare advice

I advised her not to shower for the next 24 hours so as to fully absorb the Aromatherapy oils in to her system to fully feel the benefits. The essential oils I have used will be processed and eliminated by her body within 24hours. I explained to her about making a hot compress which will help for muscular aches and pains and she said she would like to try it to see if it could help. I advised her to use one drop of lavandin or marjoram on the compress as both oils are beneficial for muscular aches and pains. I have done a patch test on my Client for Black Pepper and provided she has no irritation to the oil I will be using it next time for her muscular pain. Black pepper is a strong rubefacient oil so it produces warmth and redness when applied to the skin which will help ease the tension.

I gave my client a general homecare advice sheet outlining possible reactions and things that can help her reduce her stress level over the week.

Reflective practice

The room wasn't very warm and my client commented on it so I need to make sure to warm up the room for a good while before clients arrive. I didn't help my client off the bed when the massage was finished and it is especially important to remember to do this for safety so my client won't slip etc. I concentrated and worked longer on my clients back as this is a problem area but it meant I then went over the time I had allocated for the overall treatment. If I decided to concentrate on one area specifically in future I will reduce the amount of time I spent on other areas so I stay within the treatment time

TREATMENT 2
Reactions to last treatment

She said she slept solidly the night of the massage treatment and also the following night. She felt her stress levels for the following day were much lower and she was calmer under pressure. She felt her back was looser that night but while sitting at her desk the following day she started to feel tense and stiff again. She arrived for the appointment in that condition.

Any changes to consultation

I did a patch test on my client for Black pepper as I want to use this for muscular aches and pains. She has no adverse reactions to the oil so I will be changing Eucalyptus to Black pepper in this treatment. There are no other changes to the consultation.

Oils /Botanical Name	Drops/ Mls	Uses
Black Pepper *Piper nigrum*	3 Drops	Muscular system, aches/pains, circulatory system, stimulating, Rubefacient, coughs/colds
Marjoram *Origanum marjorana*	2 Drops	Headaches, circulation, relaxant, helps insomnia, stress, Muscular aches/pains
Neroli *Citrus Aurantium*	3 Drops	Stress relief, anxiety, insomnia, nervous system, relaxant, emotional upsets.
Sweet Almond Prunus Commmunis	25 mls	Protective, nourishing, vitamins- A, B1,B2, B6, E

Details of the treatment

I did a full body massage excluding her scalp as she was going out after the treatment. She said she had a stressful week so I decided to keep using Neroli and Marjoram. Marjoram calms and soothes an overactive mind - the brain and nervous system respond to the chemical properties of the oil once it has penetrated the body through the skin or inhalations eliciting a response- relaxing properties calm the nerves, encourage deep breathing and clear the mind. My client said she had stiff legs this week so I changed Eucalyptus to Black Pepper in this treatment as I wanted an oil that has strong rubefacient and analgesic properties. Black Pepper warms the blood bringing more oxygen nutrients to the muscles thus relieving aches and pains.

My clients thighs were very cold to touch in comparison to the rest of her legs so I spent longer doing petrissage on the Bicep Femoris, Semitendinosus and Semimembranosus muscles. Also I spent longer doing frictions around the scapulae as she had quite a few knots in these areas. I used Frictions specifically to focus on small areas of tightness around her scapulae. It is useful for releasing tension in muscles and tightness around joints.

The oils absorb into the skin to the blood- the rubefacient effects of Black pepper warm the blood so it moves faster bringing oxygen to the stiff muscles and helping to remove lactic acid and carbon dioxide. She was also stiff around the trapezius and cervical area so I worked these areas with extra petrissage movements to break down the tightness and tension there. Petrissage combined with Black pepper worked to breaks down lactic acid build up and improves blood and lymph flow. Marjoram also used in the treatment is also good when massaging tight and painful muscles as it also produces local warmth when applied to the skin, it is also an antispasmodic so it calms the nerves which tell muscles to go into spasms. When I was finished the massage I helped her to sit up and get down off the massage table.

How the client felt during the treatment

My client arrived for the appointment saying she was very tense and stiff- she had slipped twice in the week and had to walk a long distance home in the snow so she had been feeling stressed and tried. She settled quicker than first time and didn't talk much during the treatment. Her thighs were cold to touch so I did extra petrissage movements there to warm the area and increase circulation. She has cellulite here which can build up with poor circulation.

How the client felt after the treatment

She was tired at first after the treatment but started to get more alert after I gave her a glass of water to drink. She said her legs didn't feel as stiff after the treatment and she felt slightly looser around her shoulders and neck.

She hadn't done any stretches for her shoulders/ neck or made a compress for muscular aches so the massage alone wasn't going to fully solve the problem areas.

Homecare advice

I gave my client a glass of water to drink while I went through the homecare advice with her. I advised her to drink more water and try to cut down on caffeine and alcohol. She rated her stress level in work as 8 which is quite high. I asked her to look for different aspects in work that might be causing a high stress level .I think if she becomes more aware of what is causing the most stress she is in a better position to make changes.

She hadn't made any compresses this week to help alleviate her back pain; I explained to her that the massage alone would not help fully solve the problem and I suggested she tried it.

I gave her a sheet with the names of the oils I have used in the treatment and their benefits. I suggested she could use 3 drops of Bergamot in the bath if she is stressed after work to lift her spirits. Bergamot is uplifting thus reducing anger, anxiety stress and frustration.

Reflective practice

Sometimes I feel stiff when I do a massage as I tend to tense up across my shoulders and my arms. Throughout the treatment I was conscious I was doing this and I made a lot of effort to try and relax and loosen up the muscles across my back. I was slightly uncomfortable but definitely made improvements on correcting my posture. My client asked me information about the oils I used but I had to check my book as I didn't know all the details of the oils, more study is required.

TREATMENT 3
Any changes to consultation

There are no changes to the initial consultation.

Reactions to last treatment

She said she felt calmer after the massage. She wasn't aware before the massage that she was feeling tense but after the massage she felt looser. She said she felt calmer in work than usual for the next two days but started to feel agitated and frustrated in work later in the week due to her workload. She had taken on board my suggestion for putting a few drops of bergamot into her bath. This she felt had helped calm her down and lift her spirits when she started to feel stressed.

Details of the treatment

I did a full body massage leaving out the abdomen as the client doesn't like it. Her skin was very dry so I had to keep reapplying the oil. I used the same oils as the last treatment as my client liked the smells of the oils and she had a positive response to the oils after the treatment. Inhalation is the fastest way for essential oils to penetrate the body. The molecules travel up the nose the brain then picks up on the messages sending responses via the nerves around the body.

She had a few adhesions in her calf muscles- soleus and gastrocnemius. Her legs were also fairly cold to touch; the room was warm so it could suggest poor circulation. She skin reddened very quickly with the local warmth of Black pepper and Marjoram on her skin.

She said she felt tender at the cervical area of her neck. She didn't have any adhesions or stiffness in her muscles when I worked over the area but her spine was hunched at the cervical spine. It appeared to me to be more of a skeletal problem than a muscular one. This could very easily be caused by repeated poor posture and leaning instead of keeping her spine straight. Marjoram can be used for the skeletal system. The warming effects of the oil can penetrate into a joint that is normally too stiff and painful to be moved to regain some mobility. My client calmed and started to breathe much deeper by the time I started to do the face and head massages. She was holding a lot of tension in her Frontalis and Temporalis muscles. When I finished the massage I helped my client off the massage table.

How the client felt during the treatment

She talked a lot and didn't relax till near the end of the treatment. Her skin was very dry and absorbed the oil a lot quicker than usual. She said she was tender around her neck and shoulders but her muscles didn't appear to be very stiff when I worked over them with petrissage movements. There was also less adhesions here than usual.

How the client felt after the treatment

She said she felt very warm and relaxed after the treatment and felt she was tired enough to go asleep. She seemed calmer and wasn't talking as much afterwards.

Homecare advice

I gave my client a glass of water to drink. I gave her a homecare advice sheet explaining possible reactions and aftercare advice. I advised her not to shower for 24hours to give the oil time to absorb. She has a lot of upper back pain in her trapezius, rhomboids and splenius capitis muscles. I asked her last week to look out for aspects in work that are causing her stress. She doesn't look after her posture while sitting at her desk at work or do any stretches when she gets very tense.

The result is the problem gets worse and without doing daily preventive measures it doesn't improve. This leads to her feeling tired and finding it hard to concentrate on her workload. She also feels that she is often given too much work to do; she finds it hard to keep up and often has to work unpaid overtime to get the work done. I have suggested that she talks to her boss about this so that they can both come up with a solution as a high stress level can continue to affect her physical and mental wellbeing. She said she will try this week to make a hot compress. I also told her she could try 3 drops of Black pepper or Eucalyptus smithii in the bath to help with muscular aches and pains. Eucalyptus smithii will also help with relieving stress.

Reflective practice

I was much more relaxed and didn't feel as tense as the previous week. I made sure I kept my legs bent and didn't bend my back while doing the massage treatment. My client was very chatty during the treatment but I kept answering her questions and in a way kept the conversation going .I need to find a way to keep my client quite while doing the massage as It will help her relax more and I will find it easier to concentrate on the routine.

TREATMENT 4
Any changes to consultation

There are no changes to the consultation

Reactions to last treatment

She was very warm and she felt like this for the rest of the evening. She said she had a deep sleep the night of the massage and felt very relaxed for a few days after the massage. She felt her upper back muscles were still tense and sore during the week but not as bad as they had been previously. She had made a hot compress twice during the week when she had back pain and she put Black pepper oil on it, the oil is a strong rubefacient oil so it produces local warmth and redness when applied to the skin penetrating deeply into the muscles. She said she was in low spirits today but wasn't sure why she felt this way. I am using the same oils this week as the previous two weeks as she had a positive response to the previous treatment.

Details of the treatment

My client arrived for an evening treatment saying she was finding it hard relax today and was in low spirits. I performed a full body massage with emphasis on the specific areas of tension. I did extra Petrissage movements (finger rolling, thumb rolling, wringing and frictions) on her trapezius and rhomboid muscles and around her scapulae bones as this is where she was tender and had stiffness. This combined with the rubefacient effects of Black Pepper oil helped to break down lactic acid and reduce muscular aches and pains. This happens by the blood being warmed by the oil, circulation improves so there is quicker delivery of oxygen and nutrients and a faster removal of CO_2 and waste.

Neroli and Marjoram have similar properties both are used as relaxants and are stress reducing. Neroli is also specifically useful for emotional upsets and since my client was feeling low before the treatment the oil would help with this. These oils affect how the body works when they are inhaled by changing impulses and messages sent around the body. The relaxing/ distressing properties of the oils pass over the olfactory cell in the nose send messages along the nerves to the brain.

The brain then reacts to the chemicals in the oil in this case sending out messages to the body to relax such as encouraging deeper breathing, relaxing nerves and organs.

When I finished the treatment I helped my client off the massage table and gave her a glass of water to drink.

How the client felt during the treatment

My client was silent from the start of the massage and she breathed deeply .She said she felt tender around her shoulders when I worked over them. When I went to turn her over on the table she said she felt very drowsy. She was quite for the remainder of the treatment and seemed very calm at the end.

How the client felt after the treatment.

She said her mood was low before the treatment but she felt this had lifted and she felt happier after the massage. She said she felt very warm and 'cosy' also. She said she felt deeply relaxed but not fatigued. She didn't feel as much tension as usual in her upper back and shoulders.

Homecare advice

I gave my client a glass of water to drink. I talked to her again about possible reactions and aftercare advice. My client had made a hot compress during the week and had found it beneficial for her back pain so she plans to continue to do this.

I also told her she could try 3 drops Eucalyptus smithii in the bath to help with muscular aches and pains. Eucalyptus smithii will also help with relieving stress. She had put this into the bath during the week when she was feeling stressed to do with work and she felt it had really helped her to relax and unwind.

Reflective practice

I was happy with how this last treatment went, I have a lot to learn but I feel more confident my progress week to week with using the oils. My client has had good responses to the treatments and has been able to relax without discomfort during the treatments. The music went off during the treatment so next time I will remember to keep it on repeat. I had good posture this week so I didn't feel tired or sore after the treatment.

OVERALL CONCLUSION

T1: My client arrived for the first treatment with upper back tension and it was very tender. After the massage treatment she felt calmer, relaxed and sleepy. Also she felt she had less pain and tension than before the massage.

T2: Before the massage my client felt tense and stiff especially in her calf muscles, afterwards she felt tired but not as tense as before. I had given her advice the previous week to do some neck stretches and making a compress but she didn't make time to do this. I changed Eucalyptus to Black Pepper.

T3: She talked a lot and didn't relax till near the end of the massage, afterwards she said she felt relaxed and calmer. She had taken on board my suggestion for using Bergamot in the bath between the treatments to reduce her stress level and lift her spirits.

T4: Between treatments she made a hot compress to help with muscular pain. At the start of the massage she was silent then she felt drowsy towards the end of the treatment. Her mood was also low at the start of the treatment but it had lifted by the end of it.

I haven't noticed a lot of improvement to her muscular tension from week to week and she was reluctant at the start to take on board my homecare advice but once she did she had positive results to trying out the compresses and using essential oils in the bath.

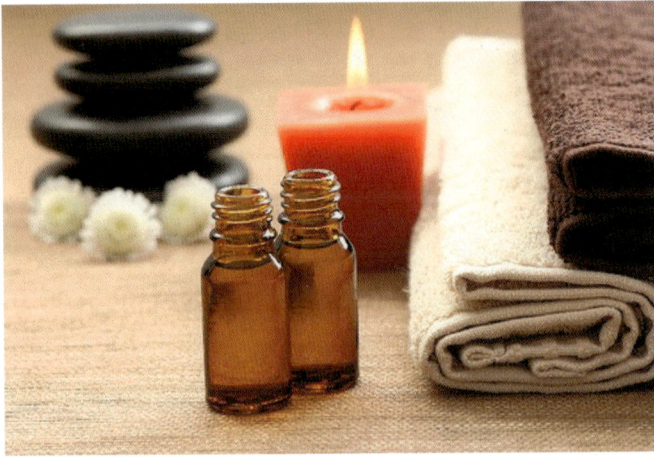

CASE STUDY 4:

Client Profile

Peter Wrenn is a full time college student in his late 20's. He is generally relaxed and good-humoured occasionally he can get very stressed due to college work. He said when he has a very heavy workload he doesn't sleep very well and it can lead to him worrying too much. He says he has had anxiety attacks occasionally over the last few years when he gets particularly stressed or when he has problems in his life but he hasn't experienced an anxiety attach for a while. He eats a healthy varied diet but he hasn't had time lately to exercise. He has no contraindications that require medical permission or restrict the treatment.

Reason for treatment

He wants a treatment to help him relax and reduce anxiety. He finds it hard to clear his mind and focus on college work and doesn't sleep well at times so he wants to try aromatherapy treatment to see if they can help with this. Relaxation, stress relief, anxiety relief and help with sleep patterns are the treatment aims. Mandarin can be phototoxic so my client needs to avoid strong sunlight and sunbeds. Juniper can irritate the kidneys so I made sure he had no kidney problems.

Rationale for the choice of each essence:

I have chosen Almond Oil for the carrier oil. This oil is easily absorbed by the skin, balances the moisture of the body and is suitable for all skin types.

I'm using Cedarwood Atlas (Cedrus Atlantica) – it reduces anxiety, tension, and stress.

Juniper (Juniperus communis) - Nervous exhaustion, Stress related disorders

Mandarin (Citrus Reticulata) – Anxiety, Insomnia, Uplifting

Treatment plan:

One Aromatherapy massage treatments every week over four consecutive weeks. It's a full body massage treatment, legs, back, scalp, arms, stomach, face and neck.

Oils Botanical Name	Drops/ Mls	Uses
Cedarwood Atlas *Cedrus Atlantica*	3 Drops	Acne, oily skin, aches and pains, stiffness, anxiety, tension, stress, cystitis, urinary tract infections, cellulite, oedema, coughs, colds
Juniper *Juniperus communis*	2 Drops	Nervous Exhaustion, stress related conditions, circulation, De-toxifying, Cellulite
Mandarin *Citrus Reticulata*	3 Drops	Anxiety, insomnia, Stomach ailments, Uplifting, refreshing, Stretch marks, oedema, Digestive
Sweet Almond *Prunus Commmunis*	25 mls	Protective, nourishing, vitamins- A, B1, B2, B6, E

TREATMENT 1
Details of how the therapist conducted the treatment

I prepared the room and the massage couch with appropriate towels. First I let my client smell the blend I used for the oils and he liked the smell, if a client dislikes particular smells they are unlikely to relax during the treatment or enjoy it. I was conscious of using oils that would be more suitable for a man so the blend had a wood and fruit aroma. I performed a Full body massage treatment. He had good muscle tone overall and didn't have any noticeable physical tension. He had a few adhesions in his gastrocnemius muscles on his left calf but no other adhesions elsewhere. The main aims of the treatment were to help him relax and reduce his stress levels. When he gets particularly stressed he finds it hard to sleep and he has had anxiety attaches previously. I chose Cedarwood Atlas for its Nervine and Sedative properties. It also has a woody sweet smell and considered to be a 'masculine' smell so it is suitable to use on men. Sedative oils reduce over-activity in the nervous system. Nervine properties strengthen and tone the nervous system.

When he inhaled the oils the molecules of the oils travel up the nose and they send messages to the brain and nerves that respond to the new smell and to the chemicals of the oils, the brain sends messages to other parts of the body to illicit a response. Sedative properties of Cedarwood atlas along with the other oils blended would cause the brain to send out messages of relaxation, calm the nerves, causing deeper breathing and mind relaxing. This was evident with the client as the more he inhaled the oils he became calmer, breathed deeper and seemed to relax fully.

When I finished the treatment I helped my client off the massage table and gave him a glass of water to drink.

How the client felt during the treatment

My client said he felt tense and wasn't relaxed before the treatment. He said he really liked the smell of the blend of the oils then he was quiet straight away and he started to breathe much deeper throughout the treatment. He didn't respond when I asked him was the pressure ok during the back massage as he had fallen asleep by this point. I had to waken him to turn him over on the table.

How the client felt after the treatment

Straight after the treatment he was fairly disorientated and he also tried to sit up straight away. I asked him to remain lying on the couch till I got him a glass of water to drink. As I suspected he was very dizzy when I helped him up to sitting so I gave him water and asked him to remain seated till he started to feel better. He said he felt totally relaxed and his mind was clearer.

Homecare advice

I asked him to drink plenty of water for the next 24 hours to help with his bodies detoxifying process. I also recommended that he left the oils on his skin for the next 24 hours if possible after the treatment to get the full benefit of the oils. I discussed possible reactions; Heightened emotions, thirst, fatigue, Skin breakouts. I explained these would pass within 24 hours if experienced and are normal reactions to treatments. I gave him a sheet with the names of the oils I have used in the treatment and their benefits. I talked to him about getting an oil burner as a method of inhaling essential oils that will help to clear his mind or for helping with sleep. Or to put two drops of essential oil onto cotton ball and place it behind the radiator in his room at night. I suggested Mandarin one of the oils I used in the treatment as it has properties to help with anxiety and insomnia.

Reflective practice

I was happy with how I conducted the treatment, I'm confident with the routine and I did the routine within time. I was also aware that my client felt disorientated afterwards and made sure to help my client up and give him a glass of water and a few minutes to become more aware of his surroundings. The room I did the treatment was very warm and I was also very thirsty during the treatment so I need to better ventilate the room next time.

Any changes to consultation

There are no changes to the consultation.

Reactions to last treatment

The night of the massage he said he slept solidly, he had no trouble going to sleep and he didn't wake up at all during the night which normally happens. He was like this for the next night also and felt a lot calmer for a few days after the treatment.

Details of the treatment

I prepared the room and the massage couch with appropriate towels. Based on my client's positive response to the last massage I decided to use the same oils again for the treatment. My client requested I left out the scalp massage this week but apart from that I performed a Full body massage treatment. He had no noticeable tension in his muscles. He had some adhesions at the top of his trapezius muscle on his left side I worked it out with extra petrissage and frictions. He said it was a bit sore when I worked over the area so I made sure not to apply too much pressure. Cedarwood atlas is good for muscular aches and pains. The oil soaks into the blood stream via the skin- it warms the blood causing it to move faster and bring more oxygen and nutrients to areas of tension and remove waste and toxins at the same time.

The main aims of the treatment were still to help him relax, reduce his stress levels and help his sleep pattern. I used Juniper as it clears and stimulates the mind and relieves stress related disorders. I choose Mandarin for its refreshing fruity aroma inhaling this oil helps to reduce anxiety and its sedative relaxing properties helps with sleep patterns, it was evident the oils had this affect with my client as at the start he was breathing quickly and he was tense and couldn't relax while lying on the table and by the end of the massage he was breathing deeper and had sunk into the table. Mandarin oil act as a depressant for the central nervous system- the oil decrease nerve impulses through the spine, brain and associated organs so as a result the person becomes more relaxed less nervous, making it easier to fall asleep and remain asleep. When I finished the treatment I helped my client off the massage table and gave him a glass of water to drink.

How the client felt during the treatment

My client chatted at the start of the treatment but he stopped after a few minutes and breathed deeply for the remainder of the treatment. He didn't fall asleep this time.

How the client felt after the treatment

He was relaxed after the treatment and he said he felt his mood had lifted. He said he didn't feel as tired as he had before the treatment but he felt calmer and more alert.

Homecare advice

I recommended again that he left the oils on his skin for the next 24 hours if possible after the treatment to get the full benefit of the oils. He said he was very tired after the last massage for that evening and the next day after the last treatment I explained this is a normal reaction to the treatment and normally would pass within 24 hours. He got an oil burner during the week and he is interested in using the oils to help with his sleep pattern and also clear his mind when he is studying. I suggested putting two drops of Mandarin and lavender into the burner with 5mls of water and putting it in his room before bedtime. Both oils have sedative relaxing properties and will help him sleep. When he is studying I have suggested he puts Peppermint into the burner to clear and focus his mind. I advised him not to burn the oil late in the evening as it refreshes the mind and would wake him up so he would find it hard to sleep.

Reflective practice

My time keeping was good this week and I was very relaxed and grounded when I did the treatment so I wasn't tense and I was able to keep the routine consistent. My client was dizzy after the last massage so I made sure to sit him up after the massage and give him a glass of water to drink and wait till I was sure he was alert enough before he got off the table. This helped and he didn't have a dizzy feeling this time. I made sure the room I performed the treatment in was better ventilated this week so it wasn't stuffy.

TREATMENT 3
Any changes to consultation

There are no changes to the consultation.

Reactions to last treatment

My client said he felt very calm after the last treatment and had felt relaxed for a few days after the treatment. He started to feel sick and run down over the last week. He was sleeping more than usual while he was feeling run down. I decided to change the oils this week to oils that would not only help with the original aims but boost his immune system also.

Oils / Botanical Name	Drops/ Mls	Uses
Peppermint / Mentha Piperita	3 Drops	Indigestion, flatulence, headaches, Cooling, Cephalic, Nervous system, Immune system
Ylang Ylang / Cananga Odorata	2 Drops	Stress reduction, Hyperventilation, Anxiety, Mental relaxant, Calming, Antidepressant, Relaxing, aphrodisiac, High Blood pressure, Palpitations.
Eucalyptus / Eucalyptus Globulus	3 Drops	Headaches, head clearing, immune system, respiratory, sinusitis, stimulating
Sweet Almond / Prunus Commmunis	25 mls	Protective, nourishing, vitamins- A,B1,B2, B6, E

Rationale for the choice of each essence:

I have chosen Almond Oil for the carrier oil. This oil is easily absorbed by the skin, balances the moisture of the body and is suitable for all skin types.

I'm using– Peppermint (Mentha Piperita) – Nervous system, Immune system, Cephalic, Refreshing.

Ylang Ylang (Cananga Odorata) - Stress reduction, mental relaxant, Calming, Anxiety.

Eucalyptus (Eucalyptus Globulus) - head clearing, Immune system.

I made sure to check my client wasn't currently using homeopathic remedies as Peppermint and Eucalyptus Globulus counteracts their benefits. Ylang Ylang can cause nausea and headaches so I only used two drops in the treatment.

Details of the treatment

I let my client smell the blend of oils and he liked the blend so I proceeded to use it. I performed a full body massage but he requested I left out the scalp on this occasion. I decided to change the blend this time as my client said he had felt run down and sick over the last week and wanted a treatment that would help boost his immune system , I was also conscious of using oils that would still help him feel relaxed and clear and focus his mind.

For reducing his stress levels I choose Ylang Ylang. This oil calms the central nervous system and is good for Stress relief and for relaxation. The oils affect how the body works by changing impulses and messages sent around the body. The relaxing/ calming properties of the oils can help to relieve symptoms of stress on the body. I choose Peppermint specifically for its Cephalic properties- it stimulates the brain and aids clear thinking. The oil clears the head, leaving the client feeling fresh and bright ready for mental effort. These molecules would be picked up by the hypothalamus which would transmit messages to the rest of the brain and body to relax, calm and settle the mind.

The properties of Eucalyptus and Peppermint also help his immune system in two ways- they can stimulate cells and organs so they are better equipped to fighting an infection and chemicals of the oils can attach bacteria already there. Peppermint is also a sudorific so it promotes sweating helping the body to eliminate toxins through the sweat glands.

How the client felt during the treatment

He chatted for a few minutes at the start of the treatment then he was much quieter and he said he didn't feel as tense after I did the back massage.

How the client felt after the treatment

He said he really liked the minty smell of the oils. He was very relaxed and he said he felt more alert and his mind was clearer.

Homecare advice

Because my client had felt sick during the week he forgot to use some of the oils in the burner. I had suggested Peppermint in the burner for clearing his mind while he is studying but it is also good for boosting his immune system so I suggested he uses this again over the week. I suggested he eats plenty of fruit and vegetables, more water and avoid alcohol to help boost his immune system and see a doctor if his symptoms persist. I gave him the remainder of the blend of oil I used in the treatment to burn in his oil burner.

Reflective practice

I was playing relaxing music during the treatment and it stopped so I need to remember to keep it on repeat next time. I was very relaxed while doing the treatment so I didn't feel tense and I kept my posture good throughout. I worked for longer on my clients back as it was tense and stiff so I needed to reduce the time that I worked on other areas.

TREATMENT 4
Any changes to consultation

There are no changes to the consultation.

Reactions to last treatment

My client said he felt relaxed for a few days after the treatment. He really liked the smell of the blend of oils and he felt physically much better after the treatment last week.

Details of the treatment

I made the same blend as last week as my client was happy for me to use it. I performed a full body massage on this occasion. I used oils that would still help him feel relaxed and clear and focus his mind. He said he felt very stressed when he arrived today for the treatment the Cephalic properties of peppermint helped to calm his mind thus reducing his stress levels. He seemed very agitated at first when he lay down on the table but after inhaling the oils for a few minutes he started to calm right down.

His back was very tense when I did effleurage and petrissage he said he hadn't don't much exercise over the last week and he felt stiff as a result. I did extra petrissage movements over the latissimus dorsi, and trapezius muscles to improve the circulation, breakdown fibrous build up and eliminate lactic acid from tension .Eucalyptus helps relieve muscular aches and pains as it has analgesic and antispasmodic properties so they will help to relieve muscular pain and it prevents and relieves spasms which can occur in tired muscles.

After the treatment he felt a bit light headed so I gave him a glass of water to drink and got him to take some deep breaths for a few minutes till he started to feel more alert.

How the client felt during the treatment

He was breathing deeply from the start of the massage and said he felt very relaxed during the treatment.

How the client felt after the treatment

My client said he had a particularly stressful day in college and he was thinking a lot but after the massage he didn't feel as agitated and his mind was much clearer.

Homecare advice

I had suggested Peppermint in the burner for clearing his mind while he is studying he used this twice over the week and he felt it helped him a lot to concentrate. I gave him the remainder of the blend of oil I used in the treatment to burn in his oil burner. My client also got Mandarin and Lavender and has put the oils in an oil burner to inhale before bedtime he finds he has been sleeping much better this week as a result and plans to continue using them. I advised him to leave on the oils for 24 hours to get the full benefit of the oils.

Reflective practice

I felt a bit tense this week also as I was stressed over having a lot of college work to do but I found inhaling the oils helped me relax also during the treatment. I felt the treatment went well I didn't rush and my client said he felt great afterwards. I had the music in the room on repeat this week so it didn't switch off in the treatment like last time.

OVERALL CONCLUSION

T1: Relaxation, stress relief, clearing/focusing his mind, anxiety relief and help with sleep patterns were the treatment aims. I chose Cedarwood atlas, Juniper and Mandarin. Before the treatment my client said he was tense, during the treatment he fell asleep. He was disorientated when he woke up. I handled the situation well by helping him up to sit, giving him water to drink and not getting him to stand up till I was sure he was more alert.

T2: After the last treatment he said he felt calmer and slept well for a few days. He was breathing quickly and wasn't relaxed at the start of the massage. During the treatment he breathed deeply and sunk into the table. Afterwards he felt his mood had lifted and he felt more alert. My time keeping was good in the treatment and I made sure my client wasn't dizzy before I got him to stand up after the treatment.

T3: My client said he felt calm and relaxed after the last treatment over the week he felt sick and run down so I changed the oils to Peppermint, Ylang Ylang and Eucalyptus. He was silent during the treatment and afterwards he said he felt relaxed, alert and his mind was clearer.

<u>T4:</u> He physically felt much better after the last treatment. He said he had a stressful day before the treatment and he was thinking a lot. During the treatment he felt relaxed and afterwards his mind was clearer.

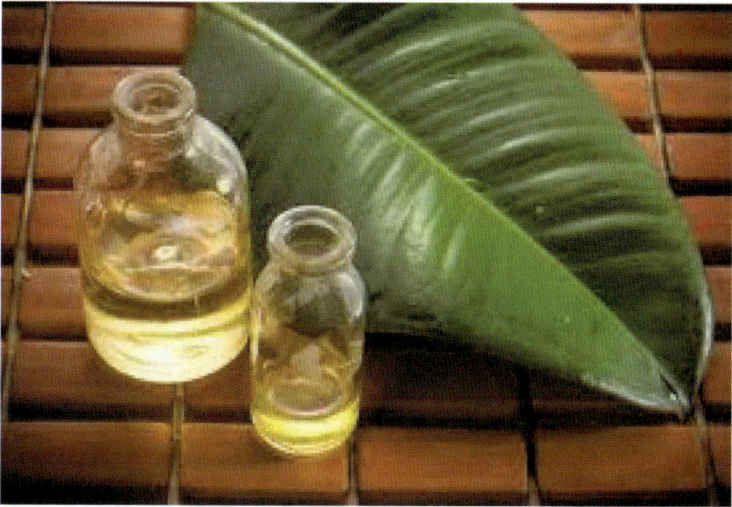

Case Study 5:

Client profile

Theresa T has come to me for Aromatherapy Treatments as personal time for her to relax. She has no Contraindications that require medical permission or Contraindications that restrict the treatment. She finds it very hard to relax and suffers from stress and depression. She feels this is due to a number of contributing factors- sedentary lifestyle, Marriage Break up, Poor Diet and workload. She finds that when she becomes stressed she suffers from tension and pain in her lower back. She said she also gets breakouts of Eczema when she is stressed. I discussed the Aromatherapy treatment in full and she has signed an informed consent form as she is happy to proceed with the treatment.

Reason for treatment: main aims of the treatment

Theresa wants a course of treatments to help her to relax. She also feels Stressed and tense and hopes aromatherapy might help with this. She also has sensitive skin so I need to use oils suitable for this.

Rationale for the choice of each essence:

Neroli- Stress Relief, very relaxing, emotional upsets, sensitive skin.

Sandalwood- Dry sensitive skin, stress,

Lavender- stress, nervous system, refreshing and relaxing.

Treatment plan:

One Aromatherapy massages every week for four weeks. I will be doing a full body massage- Legs, Back, Stomach, Arms, Face, Neck and Scalp.

Oils / Botanical Name	Drops/ Mls	Uses
Neroli / Citrus Aurantium	3 Drops	Stress relief, Anxiety, insomnia, nervous system, mature skin, Emotional Upsets, Very relaxing
Lavender / Lavandula augustifolia	3 Drops	Skincare, stress relief, relaxation, insomnia, circulation, immune system, refreshing, relaxing.
Sandalwood / Santalum album	2 Drops	Skin ailments, throat and chest infections, dry sensitive skin, Stress, depression.
Grapeseed oil / Vitis vinifera	25 mls	Smooth oil, vitamin E, no odour, linoleic acid.

TREATMENT 1

Details of how the therapist conducted the treatment

I performed a full body massage and the main emphasis of the treatment was to work on her nervous system-reducing her stress level and relaxation also I needed to incorporate in oils that are suitable for sensitive skin prone to eczema. First I let my client smell the blend of the oils, she said she liked the blend and was happy for me to proceed with it. I noticed the blend had a very weak smell but as I started to use it the smell became stronger and I found it not only relaxed my client but also relaxed me while I inhaled it. The three oils I've choose are all good for sensitive skin especially sandalwood as it is beneficial for calming irritations- the nerves and skin such as eczema. Her skin condition flares up due to stress and depression, Neroli is an antidepressant and gentle sedative. This oil has chemicals that the brain and nervous system respond to after the oil has been inhaled and penetrated into the skin, this oils properties calm and sooth the nerves, relieves stress and is an antidepressant.

The brain responds to the chemical messages and it sends out messages to the body to respond to this. In my client her response was breathing deeply, her muscles were very relaxed she felt her mind was clearer and calmer and when I talked to her at the end of the massage she was happier and her stress level had reduced. My client previously has used Lavender oil to help her get to sleep and she said she always liked the smell; this association with the oil provokes a positive response so I chose it for this reason along with its properties that support the aims of the treatment. This oil balances the emotions, lifts depression and stress. Lavender elicits responses in the same way as Neroli- influencing the brain and nervous system by changing the chemical messages sent around the body.

During the massage I didn't notice any areas of deep tension or adhesions. She did say that she felt I had relieved a lot of tension in her scalp (occipitals and frontalis) when I did the massage there, the tension build up there can be due to her stress levels.

How the client felt during the treatment

She smelt the blend and said she really liked it and from then on she inhaled the oils deeply. She was very relaxed and seemed to sink into the table and didn't move till I needed to turn her over on the table. She was drowsy at this point but said she really enjoyed the treatment so far and felt she really needed it as she had been very stressed over the last few weeks and hadn't time to relax. For the rest of the treatment she was quiet and breathed deeply. She said she liked the arm massages as she hadn't realised she was holding a lot of tension in her upper arms.

How the client felt after the treatment

After the treatment she said she felt great and she felt it helped release a lot of stress and tension she had been feeling. Her mood had lifted and she felt her mind was much clearer than what it had been before the treatment.

Homecare advice

My client felt thirsty after the treatment so I gave her water to drink. I gave her a sheet outlining general homecare advice and possible reactions. I told her not to shower for 24 hours after the treatment to get the full benefit of the oils. I discussed possible reactions; Heightened emotions, thirst, fatigue, Skin breakouts. I explained these would pass within 24 hours and are normal reactions to treatments. I gave her a sheet with the names of the oils I have used in the treatment and their benefits. I suggested she could use 3 drops of Lavender or Neroli in the bath if she is stressed to lift her spirits and relax her. She finds her biggest problem, which leads to stress, is not having much time to herself and devoting most of her time to other people. I suggested that she should try if possible to have an hour everyday where she does something that she enjoys herself that might help her relax such as a hobby or interest. I also did some deep breathing exercises with her after the treatment and I advised her to try doing ten minutes every day to see if it helps with her stress level.

Reflective practice

I was quite restricted with moving around the table so I need to allow more room next time. I hadn't much time to prepare the room as I did another treatment before this one so I need to give myself more time between them. I forgot to play relaxing music so I need to remember this for next time.

Any changes to consultation

There are some restrictive contraindications since the last treatment Bruising and cuts.

Reactions to last treatment

She said she felt great after the last massage and went home feeling refreshed. But she arrived for the appointment with very bad bruising on her right arm and cuts on her scalp and forehead. She was attacked in a row the day after the massage so she wasn't relaxed or in good form since the incident. I have decided to change Sandalwood to Rose cabbage in this treatment. This oil is non-sensitising, non-toxic, non –irritant and no known contraindications

Oils / Botanical Name	Drops/ Mls	Uses
Neroli / Citrus Aurantium	3 Drops	Stress relief, Anxiety, insomnia, nervous system, mature skin, Emotional Upsets, Very relaxing
Lavender / Lavandula augustifolia	3 Drops	Skincare, stress relief, relaxation, insomnia, circulation, immune system, refreshing, relaxing.
Rose (cabbage) / Rosa centifolia	2 Drops	Dry skin, eczema, mature/sensitive skin, uterine disorders, irregular menstruation, frigidity, PMT, depression
Grapeseed oil / Vitis vinifera	25 mls	Smooth oil, vitamin E, no odour.

Details of the treatment

My client arrived for the treatment not in great form due to being attached. I made her comfortable and before I started I established what areas I needed to leave out from the treatment. I needed to avoid her left arm, her face and her scalp this time. I decided to change Sandalwood to Rose (cabbage). I choose this oil as it stimulates positive emotions and it is a very effective anti- depressant. I let my client smell the blend before I began the treatment and she said she liked it so I proceeded to use the oils.

Rose (cabbage) has vulnerary and tonic properties so it helps wounds to heal and strengthen the body generally. She has some open cuts and bruising so I choose this oil for properties that will help this. The oil is absorbed through the surface of the skin, the hair follicles and the sweat glands they then enter the blood capillaries. When the oil reaches the blood it is transported around the whole body chemically interacting with the chemistry of her body. These properties would get to the areas affected and help with the bodies healing process.

My client has eczema at the moment on her legs this oil benefits skin conditions as it has anti-inflammatory properties and calms eczema and improves dry skin. Her eczema breaks out badly the more stressed she feels. Rose has similar properties to Lavender and Neroli used in this treatment it has anti-depressant, sedative, relaxing properties. These oils slow down activity and agitation and thus help relieve stress and tension. The affect these oils had on my client were evident when I finished the massage she was breathing much deeper, physically she appeared less tense, her shoulders were loose and she had a happy attitude.

My client had no stiffness or adhesions when I massaged over her muscles, she was tense across her shoulders but this was much looser after I worked the area with effleurage, petrissage and friction techniques. The remained of the treatment went well and no other problem areas showed up.

How the client felt during the treatment

She said she felt great during the treatment and felt she really needed it after the week she had. Her mood was low at the start of the massage but when I turned her over on the table she was breathing deeply and her expression was pleasant.

How the client felt after the treatment

She was very complimentary at the end of the massage and said she felt much better emotionally than what she had at the start and she felt it helped to relax and unwind and be pampered for a while. She was more positive and her mood had lifted at the end of the massage.

Homecare advice

I advised her not to shower for 24 hours to get the full benefit of the oils. I gave her the remainder of the blend in a container and suggested she put the oil in her burner at home for today to help her to continue to feel the benefits of the oils. I gave her the list of oils that I used and their benefits. She didn't get to put some Neroli into her bath this week but I told her to waits till the bruising and cuts have healed.

I suggested that she could put two drops of Neroli into her oil burner instead to lift her spirits and relaxation. I suggested that she tries to relax for the rest of the day and not take on anything too strenuous if possible. I gave her a glass of water and asked her to continue to drink plenty of water for the rest of the day to flush out any accumulating toxins.

Reflective practice

My client arrived for the appointment and I wasn't aware till she arrived that she had been attacked. My client explained what happened to her I said I was very sorry that this had happened. I didn't ask her any questions about it other than where exactly she had bruising and cuts so I could avoid the areas. I felt as a professional it wasn't my place to chat about the situation and that if the client wished to talk about it there would be no prompt from me and the incident would remain confidential. I was unsure whether to approach this or not in the homecare advice so I decided to stick to advice to suit the overall treatment aims of relaxation and stress reduction. My client was very pleased with the treatment and I was glad that I was able to help somewhat to lifting her mood and helping her relax.

TREATMENT 3

Any changes to consultation

There are no changes to the consultation.

Reactions to last treatment

My client was attacked before the last treatment so she had a lot of bruising and scratches. When she arrived for the treatment this week it was much improved but I decided not to do the face and head massage this week to make sure the areas were fully healed. My client was in very good spirits when she arrived and she chatted a lot. She had put some drops of Neroli into her oil burner this week and had found it beneficial for reducing her stress levels and keeping her calm. She still wanted a treatment for relaxation and she said she had aches and pains in her lower back and her arms as she was helping someone move house this week and had lifted a lot of boxes etc.

I changed Rose cabbage to Eucalyptus dives in this Treatment; I did a patch test the day before the treatment to make sure that she didn't have any reactions to the oil. She didn't have any reaction to the oil so I decided to use it to help with muscular aches and pains. It is also incompatible with homeopathic treatments so I checked my client wasn't taken any before I proceeded.

Oils / Botanical Name	Drops/ Mls	Uses
Neroli / Citrus Aurantium	3 Drops	Stress relief, Anxiety, insomnia, nervous system, mature skin, Emotional Upsets, Very relaxing
Lavender / Lavandula augustifolia	2 Drops	Skincare, stress relief, relaxation, insomnia, circulation, immune system, refreshing,
Eucalyptus / Eucalyptus dives	3 Drops	Aches pains, headaches, respiratory conditions, Expectorant
Grapeseed oil / Vitis vinifera	25 mls	Smooth oil, vitamin E, no odour, linoleic acid.

Details of the treatment

My client arrived for the treatment she was in good spirits but a bit agitated. I changed Eucalyptus to Rose Cabbage in this treatment as she had some muscular aches and pains this week. I also kept Neroli and Lavender for their stress reducing properties. I let my client smell the blend and she was happy for me to proceed to use it. My client felt her lower back was stiff when I did petrissage over the latissimus dorsi muscles. I worked the area for longer to draw more blood to the muscles to create erythema thus bring more oxygen and nutrients to the muscles. Eucalyptus is a rubefacient and an analgesic. The oil absorbs into the dermis of the skin and into the blood stream, the molecules of the oil interacts with the chemistry of her body to affect how it works. This oil warms the blood that causes vasodilation- the blood capillaries dilate so more oxygen and nutrients can get to tired muscles and there is a faster removal of waste from the tissues. The oil also has analgesic properties which reduces pain. I did palmer kneading, picking up and wringing (petrissage movements) after Effleurage.

These movements are relaxing and help to break down adhesions and reduce stiffness. My client also felt tender when I did effleurage and petrissage over her biceps and triceps. I was able to massage the arm that was badly bruised last week as it had healed. I gently massaged my client's arms checking her tolerance throughout. No other tension showed up during the treatment and she relaxed for the remainder of the massage.

How the client felt during the treatment

My client chatted a good bit at the start of the massage and although she appeared to be in good form she did seem agitated. By the time I started to work on her back I got her to do some deep breathing and she stopped talking after that and seemed much calmer. She felt tender this week when I worked on her lower back and her upper arms.

How the client felt after the treatment

After the massage my client was much calmer and breathing deeply. She said she felt great and didn't feel as tense in her lower back.

Homecare advice

I advised her not to shower for 24 hours to get the full benefit of the oils. Once again I had some of the blend left over so I gave it to her to use at home in her bath or oil burner. She had used the blend last week and said she loved it and had slept really well for a few nights afterwards. She had tension in her lower back this week so I showed her how to make a hot compress for her lower back adding one drop of marjoram to the compress. I chose this oil as it is warming for the muscles and is an analgesic and antispasmodic so it will help ease muscular aches and pains. Marjoram also helps to ease bruising which she still has on her arm so I told her she could also use the oil on the compress and put it over the bruising. I didn't advise her to do this last week as she had some cuts around the bruising but this week the cuts have healed so I think it was safe for her to do this.

Reflective practice

Last week my client had mentioned she had been attacked I feel I was professional with dealing with this and I found that this week when my client chatted she was more open again telling me things about her life. I think sometimes people feel the need to talk during treatments about their life but I feel it is best not to get involved or pass judgment or opinion on anything they say which is the way I conducted this treatment.

I was pleased with how the treatment went I kept the routine within time and kept the routine consistent and the client said she was looking forward to the next treatment so I was happy with that.

TREATMENT 4

Any changes to consultation

There are no changes to the consultation.

Reactions to last treatment

My client said she felt tired after the last treatment and she slept well that night. She felt relaxed for a few days also. The tension she had felt in her lower back was improved for a few days. She had made a hot compress with Marjoram on it and had placed it on her lower back to ease the tension.

Details of the treatment

My client arrived for an afternoon appointment and she was in a pleasant humour and looking forward to the treatment. My client was happy for me to continue using the same oils as last week. I performed a full body massage. She was calmer than usual at the start of the massage and she began to breathe deeply the longer she inhaled the oils. I still chose to use Neroli and Lavender as they are for stress relief and relaxation. Lavender combined with Neroli are depressants for the central nervous system- they decrease nerve impulses through the spine, brain and associated organs so as a result the person becomes more relaxed less nervous, making it easier to fall asleep and remain asleep.

My client was still tense in her latissimus dorsi muscles of her lower back, Eucalyptus dives is beneficial, this combined with petrissage will help reduce muscular aches and pains. I was able to apply more pressure to the muscles of her lower back this week when I was doing petrissage and thumb frictions.

When I went to massage my clients face at the end of the treatment she said she could feel tension across her forehead. I checked my client's tolerance to my pressure when I massaged across the frontalis and the temporalis muscles she felt this really helped to relax her and towards the end of the treatment she felt this tension had eased. Eucalyptus helps to ease tension headaches as it has analgesic properties. Tension across the forehead is often caused by stress and finding it hard to calm the mind and relax. Neroli and Lavender are also useful for reducing tension headaches as they have stress reducing properties that would be picked up by the hypothalamus in the brain, the brain then would send out messages to induce relaxation and calm the client. There were no other tension areas and the rest of the treatment went well.

How the client felt during the treatment

My client was very relaxed from the start of the treatment and she didn't talk much during the treatment. She said she felt tender when I did petrissage on her lower back so I used less pressure when working over the muscles.

How the client felt after the treatment

After the treatment my client said she felt great and was totally relaxed, she said she had felt tension across her forehead before the treatment but this she felt was eased afterwards. She said her back felt looser after the treatment.

Homecare advice

I advised her not to shower for 24 hours to get the full benefit of the oils. She still had tension in her lower back this week so I advised her to use the compress again to help with this. She said she felt a tension headache before the treatment so I talked to her about putting two drops of peppermint into an oil burner with water and inhaling the oil as peppermint is good for relieving headaches. I gave her a glass of water and asked her to continue to drink plenty of water for the rest of the day to flush out any accumulating toxins. I did some deep breathing exercises with her after treatment one and she has been doing this. She felt it has helped her over the last week to start of the day off feeling relaxed and calmer.

Reflective practice

I didn't have any plinth roll to cover the massage table. It looks more professional and more hygienic to have roll over the plinth cover so I will need to get some for my next treatment. I could feel myself rushing at the start of the treatment so I started to take deep breaths and do the moves slower so it would be more relaxing for my client. My client has really liked the blends I have been choosing over the last four treatments and I feel I am getting more confident in picking out blends to suit a client's needs.

.

OVERALL CONCLUSION

T1: I choose Neroli, Lavender and Sandalwood for relaxation, stress, tension and also as they are suitable for skin prone to eczema. During the treatment she was relaxed and drowsy and she felt the massage had helped to relieve tension from her scalp. After the treatment she said she felt great, less stressed and her mind was clearer.

T2: After the last treatment she said she felt great and refreshed. But my client was attacked in a row and had bad bruising and cuts. She wasn't in good humour or relaxed. I decided to change Sandalwood to Rose cabbage. She said she felt great during the treatment and afterwards she said she felt much better emotionally, relaxed and her mood had lifted. I felt as a professional it wasn't my place to comment, prompt her to talk and anything she said would remain confidential.

T3: She arrived for the treatment in a good humour and the bruising and cuts were much improved. She had used Neroli in her oil burner this week to help reduce her stress levels. She had muscular aches and pains so I changed Rose Cabbage to Eucalyptus to help with this. She seemed agitated before the treatment during it she was much calmer and after the treatment she didn't feel as tense in her lower back.

T4: She said she was relaxed for a few days after the treatment and the tension in her lower back had eased. During the treatment she felt she had tension across her forehead and her lower back was tender. She had taken on board some of my advice to use marjoram on a hot compress and the tension in her lower back wasn't as bad this week as a result.

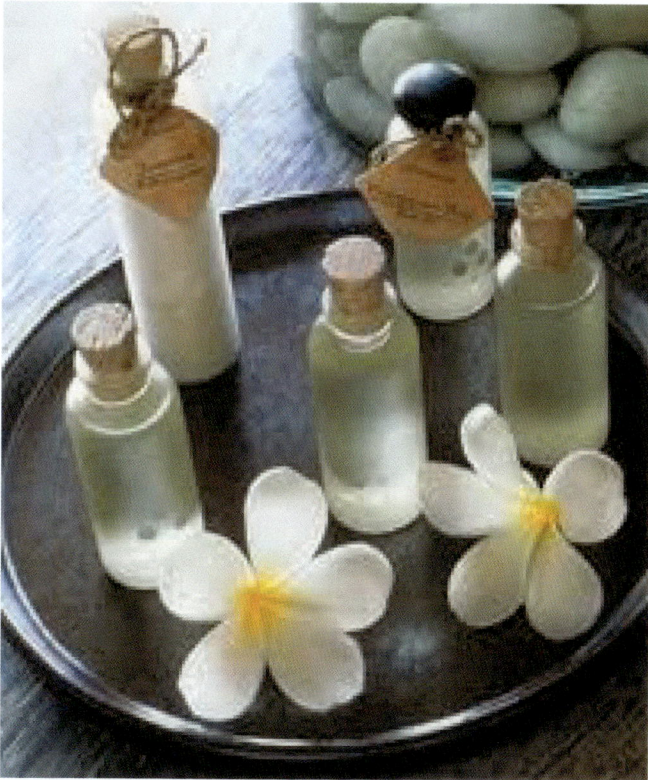

CASE STUDY: 6

Client profile

Pat C is in her 40s and she is a full time college student. She finds she is very stressed most days and she can find it hard to concentrate and relax. This leads to her feeling anxious and depressed at times.

She has had fibromyalgia around her left shoulder and this flares up depending on how stressed she feels. She is unhappy with her diet and she feels she needs to lose weight and start exercising. She has poor circulation overall and she feels this is due to lack of exercise and sedentary lifestyle. She has no contraindications that require medical permission, she has a varicose vein on the thigh of her left leg which restricts the treatment to this area.

Reason for treatment: main aims of the treatment

She has requested a treatment that will help with reducing her stress levels and aid muscular aches and pains. She can have low moods and can be anxious so I will be using oils that will also help with this.

Rationale for the choice of each essence:

Bergamot- Anxiety, Nervous tension, Uplifting.

Geranium- Circulation, Stress related conditions, Nervous tension.

Marjoram- Muscular aches and pains, Relaxant, Stress

Treatment plan:

One aromatherapy massage per week for four weeks; working on the legs, back, stomach, arms, face and head.

Oils / Botanical Name	Drops/ Mls	Uses
Bergamot / Citrus Bergamia	3 Drops	Anxiety, Depression, Nervous system, Immune system, Uplifting, Cooling.
Geranium / Pelargonium graveolens	2 Drops	Circulation, lymphatic system, anti-inflammatory, Pmt, menopause, nervous tension, stress related conditions.
Marjoram / Origanium marjorana	3 Drops	Muscular aches and pains, headaches, Circulation, Relaxant, Insomnia, and Stress.
Grape seed / Vitis vinifera	25 mls	Smooth oil, no odour, vitamin E, high in linoleic acid

TREATMENT 1

Details of how the therapist conducted the treatment

My client arrived for an afternoon appointment and before I started the treatment I let my client smell the blend she liked the blend so I proceeded to use it. The main aims of the treatment are to reduce my clients stress level and relieve muscular aches and pains. The oils I chose for this treatment are Bergamot, Geranium and Marjoram. My client was very stressed and tense when she arrived she started to relax during the treatment and breathe deeply. Bergamot is uplifting so it reduces the symptoms of stress, anxiety and depression. This I could notice in my client as after the massage the massage she was in a happier humour, calmer and more relaxed. She was also very tired and drowsy which can be a response to the sedative properties of Bergamot.

Her left shoulder was very tender when I worked around it mainly the rhomboids and the trapezius. I reduced my pressure and worked for longer around the muscles with petrissage and frictions to break down the adhesions and reduce muscular tension. I choose Marjoram as it is beneficial for muscular aches and pains.

The oil sinks into the dermis of the skin and into the blood stream. Since I worked the area for longer with petrissage there was more oxygen and nutrients brought to the tense muscles. The molecules of this oil help to warm the blood causing it to circulate better and it has properties to reduce pain. After the massage she noted that her left shoulder wasn't as painful as and less stiff than what it had been.

How the client felt during the treatment

My client was very complimentary during the treatment and felt I helped a lot to release the tension in her back. She got very drowsy while I was doing the back massage and said she still felt tired at the end of the treatment.

How the client felt after the treatment

I gave my client a glass of water to drink and it took her a few minutes to become alert. She was very happy with the massage and she said she felt deeply relaxed. She felt her left shoulder was much looser after the massage and she didn't feel in as much pain when the muscles relaxed.

Homecare advice

I told her not to shower for 24 hours after the treatment to get the full benefit of the oils. I discussed potential reactions to the treatment such as headaches, fatigue, muscular aches and pains skin reactions, bowel movements and micturition. These symptoms if experienced would quickly pass within 24-48 hours I also told her that there are many benefits to the treatments- deeper relaxation of the mind and body, increased energy levels and giving a lift to emotions increasing positive feelings. She is currently under a lot of stress due to college work it isn't necessarily the work load but her reaction to it. I suggested some positive ways of dealing with stress- walking, taking regular breaks and spending an hour every day doing a hobby or getting involved in an interest other than college work. She said she occasionally does meditation so I suggested she could try and spend 15 minutes every day doing this to see if it will help with her stress levels. I gave my client the remainder of the blend of oils to put in an oil burner today to help her relax more.

Reflective practice

I was happy with how the treatment went and I kept the treatment within the correct amount of time. I made sure to check my pressure with my client throughout and she was happy with the treatment and she found it easy to relax. I was very thirsty during the treatment and afterwards so I need to keep myself better hydrated for next time.

TREATMENT 2

Any changes to consultation

There are no changes to the consultation.

Reactions to last treatment

My client said she slept solidly the night of the massage and she said that very rarely happens. She said she felt the effect of the massage treatment for a few days afterwards- she was relaxed calmer and not as tense as usual. Later in the week she started to feel agitated again and she found it hard to concentrate.

Details of the treatment

My client arrived for the treatment saying she felt stressed and tired. She was happy for me to use the same blend as last time as she really liked the smell. My client has poor circulation and cellulite in her right thigh when I massaged over the quadriceps. I worked the area for longer with petrissage techniques to improve suppleness and break down a build up of toxins in the muscles improving the circulation. Geranium oil that I used in the treatment improves circulation and stimulates the lymphatic system so it is beneficial for reducing cellulite and improving circulation to the area.

The oil seeps into the dermis of the skin where it enters to bloodstream. The oil molecules are transported all around the body interacting with the body's chemistry to create a desired effect. In this case geranium stimulates the blood flow so oxygen nutrients get to muscles quicker and toxins are removed quicker. Stimulating blood flow and the lymphatic system helps in eliminating cellulite, which is a lumpy deposit of body fat and stimulated the removal of waste in the lymphatic system. I chose Geranium mainly as it is a tonic for the nervous system, it lifts the spirits relieves anxiety and stress. Her stress levels were high when she arrived for the treatment and she said she felt agitated. After inhaling the blend of oils during the treatment she became calmer and more relaxed by the end of the treatment. Her shoulder was still tender this week but not as stiff as the last time I worked around it. I was able to apply more pressure when I did petrissage around the rhomboids and the trapezius muscles.

How the client felt during the treatment

I checked my pressure with my client while I was doing frictions around her left shoulder this side was tenderer than the right side so I needed to reduce my pressure with the movements. I did petrissage for longer around the muscles on this side to cause erythema. She said she felt very relaxed and she really liked my massage routine.

How the client felt after the treatment

After the treatment my client was very tired and it took her a few minutes to become alert and sit up. She said she felt very thirsty after the treatment and she drank the water very quickly. She said she felt dizzy so I got her to sit up slowly and asked her to breathe deeply for a few minutes till this passed. She said she didn't feel as stiff and tense as she had been before the massage.

Homecare advice

I discussed possible reactions with my client last week and she hadn't experienced any and she had positive results to the treatment feeling deeply relaxed and sleeping well. She felt the benefits for a few days then she started to worry too much and started to feel anxious.

This led to her feeling stressed and her fibromyalgia flared up. I suggested some oils this week to help calm her- basil as it is uplifting and clears and focuses the mind and grapefruit as it is refreshing and uplifting to relieve stress. I told her she could put two drops of each into her oil burner with 10mls of water when she feels particularly stressed and not able to concentrate. She said that she would try my suggestion over the week. She had made some time twice this week to go for a walk and she felt invigorated and not as stressed afterwards so she is planning to go regularly in future. For her Fibromyalgia I suggested she tries to make a hot compress. The compress would need to be soaked in 100mls of water and one drop of Rosemary and put the compress over the affected area. Rosemary is beneficial for muscular aches and pains.

Reflective practice

My client was very complimentary about the massage and I was glad it helped her relax. I spent longer working around her shoulders during this treatment and I didn't shorten the massage to compensate for this so I went over the time, I need to cut back on other areas if I decided to work longer on one area next time.

TREATMENT 3

Any changes to consultation

There are no changes to the consultation

Reactions to last treatment

She had the same experience as last week in that she slept really well that night and for a few days she was much calmer. She also felt her mood was lifted and she was in better humour. My client had a cough and cold this week when she arrived for the treatment and she said she felt physically run down.

Oils / Botanical Name	Drops/ Mls	Uses
Bergamot / Citrus Bergamia	3 Drops	Anxiety, Depression, Nervous system, Immune system, Uplifting, Cooling.
Geranium / Pelargonium graveolens	2 Drops	Circulation, lymphatic system, anti-inflammatory, Pmt, menopause, nervous tension, stress related conditions.
Cedarwood Atlas / Cedrus Atlantica	3 Drops	Aches and pains, anxiety tension, stress, cystitis, urinary tract infections, cellulite ,oedema, coughs , colds, catarrh, bronchitis
Grape seed / Vitis vinifera	25 mls	Smooth oil, no odour, vitamin E, high in linoleic acid

I changed Marjoram to Cedarwood atlas in this blend my client said she felt run down when she arrived and she had a cold and chesty cough. I still needed to choose oils that would benefit her initial aims also of stress relief and muscular aches and pains. Cedarwood atlas is non-toxic and non-sensitising so it is safe to use without a patch test.

Details of the treatment

When I was ready to begin the massage I left my client smell the blend and she was happy to proceed with it. I changed Marjoram in the blend to Cedarwood Atlas. I chose Cedarwood Atlas for its Nervine and Sedative properties. Sedative oils reduce over-activity in the nervous system. These properties strengthen and tone the nervous system. When she inhaled the oils the molecules of the oils travel up the nose and they send messages to the brain and nerves that respond to the new smell and to the chemicals of the oils, the brain sends messages to other parts of the body to illicit a response. Sedative properties of Cedarwood atlas along with the other oils blended would cause the brain to send out messages of relaxation, calm the nerves, causing deeper breathing and mind relaxing. This was evident with the client as the more she inhaled the oils she became calmer, breathed deeper and seemed to relax fully.

Cedarwood atlas is good for muscular aches and pains. The oil soaks into the blood stream via the skin- it warms the blood causing it to move faster and bring more oxygen and nutrients to areas of tension and remove waste and toxins at the same time. Her trapezius muscles and rhomboids were tense again this week but I was able to apply more pressure when doing frictions and petrissage over the muscles.

My client had a chesty cough and a cold and she said she felt physically run down. This oil is good for the respiratory system. It is a Mucolytic and an Expectorant so it breaks down catarrh in the nose and respiratory passages and helps fluidity thus removing mucus from the lungs and respiratory passages. The oil is inhaled through the nose and the chemical molecules react with the chemistry of the body and start to create the desired effect in this case clearing up mucus and reducing it helping the virus to clear up quicker. My client found it hard to breathe while lying face down on the table and she was very congested. When I was working on her face at the end of the treatment I spent longer sweeping my fingers from the sides of the nose out towards the submandibular and auricular nodes to help clear out the mucus and infection. She found it much easier to breathe after this and she didn't feel as congested after the treatment.

How the client felt during the treatment

My client moved a bit on the table at the start of the massage and she found it hard to relax. She said she had a stressful day and didn't feel very calm. Her sinuses were congested and she had a cough and cold so she didn't find it easy to breathe while lying face down. After a few minutes she started to settle and she was relaxed for the rest of the treatment.

How the client felt after the treatment

After the treatment she said she felt very calm and that her mind was much clearer than what it had been at the start of the massage. She was breathing much deeper and clearer. She wasn't coughing as much after the treatment. She said overall she felt really good and complimented me on the treatment.

Homecare advice

My client tried my suggestion for putting grapefruit and basil in her oil burner this week she felt much more relaxed as a result and her mind was clearer she said she plans to keep using this in future. She didn't make a compress this week for her back as she didn't have time but she felt it wasn't as bad this week. Today when she arrived for the treatment she said she felt very stressed and agitated, she was calmer after the massage but I suggested she tries to do some meditation or go for a walk this evening to help clear her head. I suggested steam inhalation to help with her respiratory system. I made a blend of Benzoin (its soothing for her throat), Cedarwood and Eucalyptus globulus. The blend could be put into a basin of hot water and inhaled while covering her head with a towel for several minutes. I made her enough to use for a few days.

Reflective practice

My client found it very hard to relax at the start of the massage so I did the massage techniques slowly and lightly which helped her relax. I was able to apply more pressure this week while working over my clients shoulder and I made sure to check my client's tolerance to my pressure. I wasn't very relaxed this week doing the treatment and was tense across my shoulders I tried to keep breathing deeply and loosening my arms instead of tensing them and it seemed to help.

TREATMENT 4

Any changes to consultation

There are no changes to the consultation

Reactions to last treatment

She said she was very calm that day when she went home after the massage. The next day she had nausea and a headache but she wasn't sure if this was related to the massage. She slept really well for a few days but started to feel stressed and had a low mood when she went back to college later in the week. She felt her respiratory system was much better she felt the cold was nearly gone and she wasn't coughing as much, she said she was still bringing up a lot of mucus. She had used the blend over the last week for inhalation and she felt it had really helped her feel better.

Details of the treatment

After talking with my client I decided to use the same blend of oils this week, she was nearly over her cough and cold but still had a lot of mucus so I decided to keep using the Cedarwood for this purpose. Also her stress level is still high and she had a low mood so I decided to keep using the bergamot and geranium to help with this.

My client's lower back was tense this week when I worked over the latissimus dorsi and the external obliques when I did petrissage. The muscles here were also much colder to work over which could suggest poor circulation. I did extra Petrissage movements (finger rolling, thumb rolling and this combined with Cedarwood atlas oil helped to break down lactic acid and reduce muscular aches and pains. This happens by the blood being warmed by the oil, circulation improves so there is quicker delivery of oxygen and nutrients and a faster removal of CO_2 and waste. I checked throughout with my client to make sure I was applying the right amount of pressure. My client was still tender in her upper back around the rhomboids/ trapezius on her left side which is where she has the fibromyalgia I worked the tension with light pressure doing frictions and petrissage checking my clients tolerance. When I had finished the massage I helped my client off the massage table and gave her a glass of water to drink.

How the client felt during the treatment

My client chatted for the first few minutes but she relaxed quickly and started to breathe deeply. She said she hadn't slept well the night before and felt she was in low spirits for the last few days.

The tension in her left shoulder was much worse today and she felt this was due to doing a lot of treatments this week and being stressed over college work.

How the client felt after the treatment

At the end of the treatment her mood had lifted. She appeared calmer. Her shoulders had dropped and she didn't seem as hunched as what she had at the start. She said she felt deeply relaxed but not drowsy like previous weeks.

Homecare advice

After the last massage my client didn't feel well the next day with nausea and a headache. I explained not to be alarmed if this happens just drink plenty of water to flush out accumulating toxins and try and rest as much as possible. I talked to her about her stress levels in relation to college that having a high stress level regularly can have a negative effect on her for example leading to depression, insomnia, chest pains and make her fibromyalgia worse for instance. I suggested she should try to do deep breathing when she feels like that and not concentrate on negative thoughts and breaking her work load down into manageable chunks can help her get through the workload efficiently. She didn't get to use the oils this week in the burner but she plans to continue to use them when she is stressed and needs to concentrate.

Reflective practice

I worked for longer around my clients shoulders again this week and she said she felt great afterwards so I was pleased with how the treatment went. I made sure to keep the treatment within the right time this week so was pleased with that. I applied a bit too much oil to my client's arms I need to apply less next time as my hands slid a bit with the oil.

OVERALL CONCLUSION

T1: I chose Bergamot, Geranium and Marjoram to help with reducing her stress levels and aid muscular aches and pains. She was stressed when she arrived. During the treatment she was drowsy. After the treatment she felt deeply relaxed and her left shoulder was much looser where she has Fibromyalgia.

T2: After the last treatment she slept solidly and she was relaxed and calmer. She also didn't feel as tense as usual. She felt agitated later in the week and her left shoulder was tense. After the treatment she was thirsty and felt a bit dizzy. She had less muscular tension and she felt tired.

T3: My client slept really well after the last massage and she was much calmer for a few days. She had a cough and a cold when she arrived so I changed Marjoram to Cedarwood Atlas as the oil is beneficial for this. After the massage she said her mind was clearer, she felt calmer and she didn't feel as congested and she coughed less.

T4: After the last massage she felt calm that day. The next day she had a headache and nausea. I made a blend the previous week for her to inhale to help with her cough and cold and she felt it had helped to ease it. She said she was feeling low the last few days and her mood had lifted, she was calmer and more relaxed after the massage.

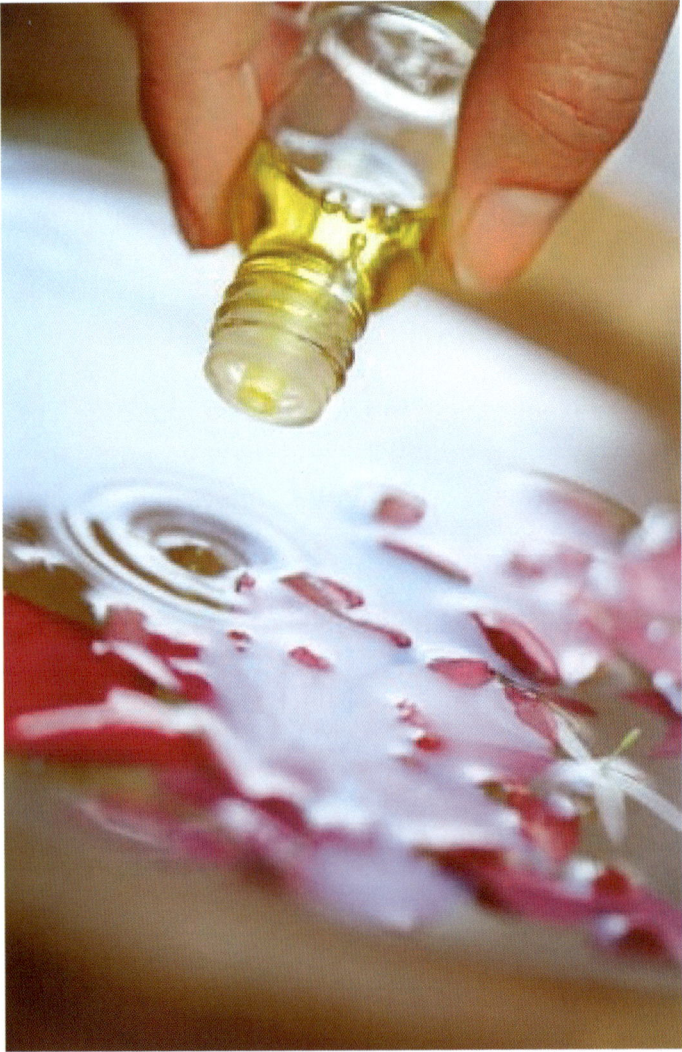

CASE STUDY 7:

Client profile

Lilly D is 25 years old and a full time College student. She is very busy with college work and doesn't have much time to relax and unwind at the moment. She has a varied healthy diet but doesn't get time to exercise as much as she would like. Occasionally she can be stressed due to her college work but in general she is in good spirits and tries not to get overwhelmed by her workload. She doesn't sleep well at times which can be due to when she is stressed, works late and she also drinks a lot of coffee. She has no Contraindications that require medical permission or Contraindications that restrict the treatment. I discussed the Aromatherapy treatment in full and she has signed an informed consent form as she is happy to proceed with the treatment.

Reason for treatment: main aims of the treatment

The main aim of the treatment is helping the client to relax and unwind. She finds it hard to clear and focus her mind when she is studying and when she gets particularly stressed she doesn't sleep well. I have chosen Grapeseed Oil for the carrier oil. This oil is smooth so it is good for a Full Body Massage, it also has no odour so it doesn't influence the smell of blend. I've chosen Peppermint, Neroli and Ylang Ylang for this treatment.

Rationale for the choice of each essence:

Peppermint (Mentha Piperita) - Cephalic; Clears and focuses the mind, Nervous system

Neroli (Citrus Aurantium) - Stress relief, Nervous System, Relaxing

Ylang Ylang (Cananga Odorata) - Positive emotions, Calming and Relaxing

I checked the safety factor with my client peppermint is not compatible with homeopathic treatments. Neroli has no known and Ylang Ylang can cause headaches and nausea so needs to be used in moderation.

Treatment plan:

One aromatherapy massage per week for four weeks ; working on the legs, back, stomach, arms, face and head.

Oils / Botanical Name	Drops/ Mls	Uses
Peppermint / Mentha Piperita	3 Drops	Indigestion, Headaches, Cooling, refreshing,cephalic,nervous system, Immune system
Neroli / Citrus Aurantium	3Drops	Stress relief, Nervous System, Relaxing, Anxiety, Insomnia, Eases palpatations
Ylang Ylang / Cananga Odorata	2 Drops	Positive emotions, Calming and Relaxing, Euphoric Effect, Aphrodisiac
Grapeseed Oil / Vitis Vinifera	25 mls	Vitamin E, finely textured, Linoleic Acid

TREATMENT 1

Details of how the therapist conducted the Treatment

First I let my client smell the blend of oils I mixed and she didn't like the smell, if a client dislikes particular smells they are unlikely to relax during the treatment or enjoy it. The oils I choose first were Peppermint, Neroli and Vetiver. Vetiver dominated the other smells in the blend and it was quite potent so I changed the blend then to Peppermint, Neroli and Ylang Ylang. She liked this blend better so I proceeded to do a full body massage with emphasis on the specific areas of tension. I did extra Petrissage movements (finger rolling, thumb rolling, wringing and frictions) on her trapezius and rhomboid muscles and around her scapulae bones as this is where she had a lot of tension and adhesions. She asked me to leave out the face and head massage as she doesn't like being massaged there. I choose Peppermint specifically for its Cephalic properties- it stimulates the brain and aids clear thinking. The oil clears the head, leaving the client feeling fresh and bright ready for mental effort.

These molecules would be picked up by the hypothalamus which would transmit messages to the rest of the brain and body to relax, calm and settle the mind. I made sure to check my client wasn't currently using homeopathic remedies as Peppermint counteracts their benefits.

Neroli and Ylang Ylang have some similar properties both are used for Stress relief and for relaxation. These oils affect how the body works by changing impulses and messages sent around the body. The relaxing/ calming properties of the oils can help to relieve symptoms of stress on the body. Ylang Ylang can cause nausea and headaches so I only used two drops in the treatment. When I finished the treatment I helped my client off the massage table and gave her a glass of water to drink.

How the Client felt during the treatment

My client was tired from the start of the treatment. During the treatment she got very drowsy and she fell asleep. She started to wake up when I went to turn her over on the table.

How the client felt after the treatment

At the end of the treatment she said she felt very calm and her mind was cleared. I gave her a glass of water to drink and let her relax for a while before getting off the couch and putting her shoes back on. She said she enjoyed the treatment and was interested to see how the treatments would progress. The next treatment will be in a weeks' time.

Homecare advice

I advised my client not to shower for the next 24 hours to absorb the oils and get the benefits. I gave my client a glass of water to drink while I went through the homecare advice with her. I advised her to drink more water and try to cut down on caffeine and alcohol. I discussed possible reactions; Heightened emotions, thirst, fatigue, Skin breakouts. I explained these would pass within 24 hours and are normal reactions to treatments. I gave her a sheet with the names of the oils I have used in the treatment and their benefits. I suggested she could put two drops of Peppermint into an Oil burner with a small amount of water when she is trying to study. Peppermint is a cephalic so it clears and focuses the mind and it will help her to concentrate when she is studying.

Reflective practice

I was careful to watch my posture during the treatment so as not to bend my back, the massage table was lower than I usually have it so I needed to bend my knees more. I also have to watch my breathing as at times I can hold my breath during the treatment without realising.

TREATMENT 2

Any changes to the consultation

There are no changes to the consultation.

Reactions to the last treatment

My client said she felt calm after the last treatment for the rest of the evening; she also was very tired and thirsty for the rest of the day. I explained that feeling this way can be a possible short-term reaction to a treatment that will pass. She put some peppermint into her oil burner a few times this week to help focus her mind when she was studying and she found it beneficial. She felt her mood was low the last few days and she wasn't sleeping very well which was leading to her feeling more stressed.

I decided to change the oils in this treatment, in this case study I want to try out different blends but sticking to the overall aims of relaxing the client.

Oils / Botanical Name	Drops/ Mls	Use
Neroli / Citrus Aurantium	3 Drops	Stress relief, Nervous System, Relaxing, Anxiety, Insomnia, Eases palpatations
Bergamot / Citrus Bergamia	3 Drops	Anxiety, Depression, Nervous system, Immune system, Uplifting, Cooling.
Basil / Ocimum Basilicum	2 Drops	Antiseptic, Antispasmodic, Headaches, Uplifting refreshing, Digestion, cephalic, tonic.
Jojoba / Simmondsia chinensis	25 mls	Finely textured, nourishing, useful for many skin conditions, suitable for all skin types, fatty acids- erucic, palmitic and palmitoleic acids.

Rational for the choice of each essence:

Neroli - stress relief, insomnia, relaxing

Bergamot - anxiety, uplifting.

Basil - cephalic, uplifting, insomnia, stress.

Jojoba- finely textured, suitable for all skin types.

Neroli has no known safety factors, Bergamot can be phototoxic so I advised my client to avoid strong sunlight and sunbeds. Basil needs to be avoided during pregnancy and my client isn't pregnant so it is safe to use on her.

Details of how the therapist conducted the treatment

My client arrived for an afternoon appointment I decided to try another blend of oils that still fit my clients aims of relaxation, clearing her mind, stress and sleep problems. My client smelt the blend of oils and she was happy for me to proceed with the blend. I chose Basil, Bergamot and Neroli.

Bergamot is uplifting so it reduces the symptoms of stress, anxiety and depression. This I could notice in my client as before the massage she had a low mood and after she was more positive, calmer and more relaxed. She was also very tired and drowsy which can be a response to the sedative properties of Bergamot.

Neroli is also a gentle sedative, stress reliever and helps with sleep problems. This oil has chemicals that the brain and nervous system respond to after the oil has been inhaled and penetrated into the skin, this oils properties calm and sooth the nerves, relieves stress and is an antidepressant. The brain responds to the chemical messages and it sends out messages to the body to respond to this.

She started to relax fully when I massaged the splenius capitis, sternocleidomastoid, and the occipitalis muscles. Massaging her scalp and neck combined with the properties of these oils helps to stimulate the parasympathetic nervous system which helps to promote rest, relaxation, sleep and stress reduction. The remainder of the treatment went well and my client was able to relax fully.

How the client felt during the treatment

My client seemed agitated at the start and her mind wasn't focusing on relaxing and I could feel the tension in her body. She was starting to get relaxed when I massaged her scalp and back of her neck. She relaxed quickly when I turned her over on the table.

How the client felt after the treatment

She felt light headed after the treatment so I gave her a glass of water to drink and got her to breathe deeply for a few minutes till she felt more alert then I helped her down off the table. She said she felt positive and uplifted and her mind was clearer.

Homecare advice

After the last treatment my client felt thirsty and tired which I explained can be a possible reaction that often passes in 24 hours. I advised her to respond to her bodies requirements for rest etc. and drink plenty of water which helps relieve the symptoms. I had some of the blend left over the treatment which she could put into her bath or into her oil burner this evening after the treatment. She used Peppermint in her oil burner to help focus her mind to study but I advised her not to burn the oil too late in the evening as it is a stimulant and she could find it hard to sleep as it can make a person very alert. I advised her to put two drops of lavender or chamomile into her oil burner before bed to help her sleep. My client said her workload is now getting harder and she is getting more stressed so I suggested she tries to take regular breaks when she is studying and some light exercise such as walking or yoga can help her bring down her stress levels.

Reflective practice

I was happy overall with how the treatment went, my client started to relax during the treatment and she said she enjoyed it. I will try to help my client to relax next time before the treatment starts by getting the client to do deep breathing exercises to calm them. My nails were a bit long in this treatment I need to remember to have them shorter next time for hygiene purposes. I watched my posture throughout the treatment to make sure I didn't hunch or strain myself during it.

TREATMENT 3

Any changes to the consultation

There are no changes to the consultation.

Reactions to the last treatment

My client felt alert and relaxed after the last treatment which she liked as she still had a lot of college work to do when she went home after the treatment. She felt her mind was clearer and she was able to get on with her workload. She still has used peppermint in her oil burner in the evenings and she found she is finding it easier to settle into her workload and getting through it much more efficiently. Towards the end of the week she was feeling particularly stressed and didn't sleep well for a few nights. She finds she can get stressed then from worrying if she will be able to get to sleep at night or not. My client said she liked the oils I used last week but was interested to try another blend and I was happy to do this as I want to gain more experience of mixing different blends that are still suitable for the aims of the treatment.

Rational for the choice of each essence:

Geranium-, Stress related conditions, Nervous tension.

Sandalwood- stress, relaxing, sedative.

Basil- Cephalic, uplifting, insomnia, stress.

Oils / Botanical Name	Drops/ Mls	Use
Geranium / Pelargonium graveolens	3Drops	Tonic, uplifting, stimulant, nervous tension, stress related disorders, circulatory problems, oedema.
Sandalwood / Santalum album	3 Drops	Antidepressant, antispasmodic, antiseptic, relaxing sedative, tonic.
Basil / Ocimum Basilicum	2 Drops	Antiseptic, Antispasmodic, Headaches, Uplifting refreshing, Digestion, cephalic, tonic.
Jojoba / Simmondsia chinensis	25 mls	Finely textured, nourishing, useful for many skin conditions, suitable for all skin types, fatty acids- erucic, palmitic and palmitoleic acids.

Details of how the therapist conducted the treatment

My client arrived for a morning appointment and I changed the blend. My client smelled the blend when it was prepared and said she was happy for me to use it. She was a bit restless and didn't seem very comfortable till I was a few minutes into the massage routine. I used Basil as it is a cephalic the oil is inhaled and is picked up by the olfactory membranes at the top of the nose. Once these membranes are triggered by the oil these send messages along the olfactory nerves to the brain, the brain then responds to the molecules. This oil has molecules that clear and focus the mind making the brain more efficient and alert this in turn helps to reduce the client's agitation and helps her to relax.

I chose Geranium and Sandalwood as they are a tonic for the nervous system, relieving anxiety and stress. My client was agitated and stressed when she arrived for the treatment and inhaling the blend of oils during the treatment she became calmer and less anxious. Sandalwood and Basil are both good for sleep problems which my client experiences due to stress. Basil would clear and focus the mind and Sandalwood would help to relax and sedate her which would make it easier for her to be able to go to sleep and stay asleep.

I did a full body massage on my client her areas of tension were the latissimus dorsi, the rhomboids and the trapezius muscles this seemed more stress related as when she started to relax the tension of the muscles started to ease and she seemed to sink more into the table while I worked over the area with effleurage and petrissage.

How the client felt during the treatment

She was a bit restless at the start of the massage and I got her to do some deep breathing exercises for a few minutes till she relaxed when I started the treatment. She was very tense when I worked on her back but towards the end of the back massage she started to sink into the table and she was still this way for the remainder of the treatment.

How the client felt after the treatment

When my client arrived for the treatment she said she was worrying and anxious about her college studies, she felt her mind was much calmer after the treatment and she wasn't stressing out as much. She said she felt relaxed but still alert after the treatment.

Homecare advice

I gave her a glass of water after the treatment and I advised her to continue to drink plenty of water for the rest of the day to help flush out toxins. She has started to cut down on coffee and she finds burning the peppermint oil helps keep her alert and focused instead. She didn't sleep well this week and had forgotten to burn lavender or chamomile but she plans to try it this week if she is having sleeping problems. She took regular breaks a few days this week when she was sitting in front of the computer typing college work she found her eyes didn't strain as much and she didn't feel as stiff afterwards so she plans to continue doing this. She has found she is in a low mood when she is under pressure and doesn't sleep well so I suggested she could put two drops of bergamot oil onto a cotton wool ball and place it on or behind a radiator when it is on. The heat from the radiator evaporates the oil and the aroma circulates the room.

Reflective practice

I spent a few minutes at the start of the massage doing deep breathing exercises with my client which helped her relax much more from the start of the treatment. My client has tried out some of my homecare suggestions and she is getting positive results so I am happy that she is responding well and willing to try out what I recommend. I felt myself rushing when I was doing the arm massages as I was starting to feel tired but I started to breathe more deeply ,relax my body more and slow down the movements to make the treatment more relaxing for my client. Overall I felt the treatment went well and my client enjoyed it.

Any changes to the consultation

There are no changes to the consultation.

Reactions to the last treatment

My client had a busy few days after the last treatment she kept herself focused on the work by burning peppermint and taking regular breaks from her studies. She also burned some lavender in her oil burner at night and she found it helped her sleep better than usual. So she has been happy with how the oils have helped her over the last week. She arrived today saying she felt tense and stiff she has been to the gym yesterday and felt she over did it and also she has felt on edge as it is leading up to her mock exams. I changed Sandalwood to Cedarwood Atlas in this treatment the client had muscular aches and pains and stiffness, I also chose this oil as it is for anxiety and tension. Cedarwood atlas needs to be avoided during pregnancy but other than that it has no other safety factors.

Oils / Botanical Name	Drops/ Mls	Use
Geranium / Pelargonium graveolens	3Drops	Tonic, uplifting, stimulant, nervous tension, stress related disorders, circulatory problems, oedema.
Cedarwood Atlas / Cedrus Atlantica	3 Drops	Aches, pains, stiffness, anxiety, tension , stress, cellulite, oedema, coughs, colds, catarrh, bronchitis.
Basil / Ocimum Basilicum	2 Drops	Antiseptic, Antispasmodic, Headaches, Uplifting refreshing, Digestion, cephalic, tonic.
Jojoba / Simmondsia chinensis	25 mls	Finely textured, nourishing, useful for many skin conditions, suitable for all skin types, fatty acids- erucic, palmitic and palmitoleic acids.

Details of how the therapist conducted the treatment

My client had muscular aches and pains when she arrived for the treatment so I changed Sandalwood to Cedarwood. This oil also has Nervine and Sedative properties. Sedative oils reduce over-activity in the nervous system and Nervine properties strengthen and tone the nervous system. This oil combined with the other oils blended would cause the brain to send out messages of relaxation, calm the nerves, causing deeper breathing and mind relaxing.

I checked the tolerance of my pressure while I did petrissage on my clients back. She was tender at her lower back at the Latissimus Dorsi and External obliques. I massaged the area for longer to cause erythema- warming the muscles and drawing more blood to the tissues. Cedarwood Atlas soaks into the blood stream via the skin- it warms the blood causing it to move faster and bring more oxygen and nutrients to areas of tension and remove waste and toxins at the same time. Her trapezius muscles and rhomboids were tense also but I was able to apply more pressure when doing frictions and petrissage over the muscles and they seemed to ease by the end of the treatment. She felt her arms were very achy before the treatment and she said she especially liked the arm massages this week as they were less tense afterwards.

How the client felt during the treatment

My clients back and arms were tense when I massaged them. I did the moves slowly and checked my pressure with my client she was tender at her rhomboids and trapezius muscles and she had some adhesions there that I needed to spend longer working them out. She started to relax more after I turned her over on the table and she started to fall asleep towards the end of the treatment.

How the client felt after the treatment

After the treatment she said she felt her back and her arms were much looser and overall she didn't feel tense physically or mentally. She said she felt very calm and relaxed and she was in a good humour after the treatment.

Homecare advice

I gave her a glass of water after the treatment and I advised her to continue to drink plenty of water for the rest of the day to help flush out toxins. She burned some lavender in her oil burner this week and it helped her sleep better so she plans to continue to use this. She had muscular aches and pains this week so I made a blend of Cedarwood atlas and Eucalyptus Smithii with Grapeseed oil that I advised her to put into her bath at home to help ease muscular aches and pains as both oils have properties to help with this.

Reflective practice

I had good time keeping in this treatment I spent a bit longer working on my clients arms and back so I reduced the time elsewhere to keep within the time. I breathed deeply during the treatment and I found inhaling the oils helped me relax also. My client was very pleased with the treatment and I was happy that she has been able to relax in the treatments and enjoy them. I feel I am getting more confident with picking out oils that are best suited to my client's needs and I am starting to know the oils well and explain their benefits confidently to my client.

CONCLUSION

T1: I chose Peppermint, Neroli and Ylang Ylang for this treatment. I chose these oils as my client wants a treatment that will relax, clear and focus her mind, she doesn't sleep well and she is often stressed. During the treatment she was tired, drowsy and she fell asleep. After the treatment she was calmer her mind was clearer and she said she enjoyed the treatment.

T2: After the last treatment she was tired thirsty but felt calmer. She put peppermint into her oil burner like I suggested and it help her while she studied. When she arrived her mood was low she wasn't sleeping well and she was stressed. I changed the blend of oils to Neroli, Bergamot and Basil. At the start of the massage she felt agitated and she wasn't relaxed after I massaged her scalp she started to relax. After the treatment she felt positive, uplifted and slightly light headed.

T3: In response to the last treatment she felt relaxed, alert, her mind was clearer and she was able to get on with her workload. I changed this blend to Geranium, Sandalwood and Basil. She felt restless during the treatment and tense when I worked on her back, afterwards her mind was clearer and she was calmer and not as stressed.

T4: Between the treatments she took on board my recommendation s to burn peppermint to focus her mind and lavender to help her sleep and she found they helped. She changed Sandalwood to Cedarwood to help with my client's muscular aches and pains. During the treatment my clients back and arms were tense, she relaxed and nearly fell asleep towards the end of the treatment. Afterwards she felt loose and didn't feel physically tense and she was calmer and more relaxed and in a good humour.

I changed my blend in every treatment but still stuck to the aims of the treatment of helping her to relax, clear her mind and help with her sleep problem. She responded to the blends I chose and the desired effects were achieved she was also willing to try out my suggestions in homecare advice every week and she found the oils I suggested helped her.

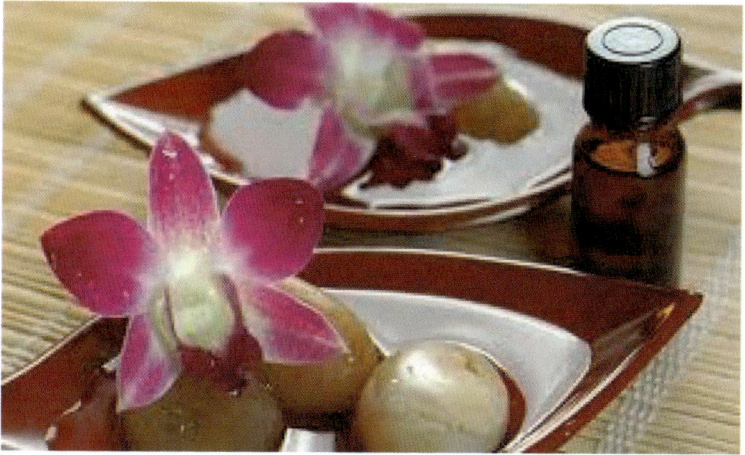

CASE STUDY 8

Client profile

Kathy W is in her 40s and is married with two children. She is attending college three days a week and also working as a complimentary therapist outside college. At the moment she feels she has fatigue due to having so much work to do between college, work and raising a family. She said she gets a tense neck and shoulders due to the nature of her work and she has poor circulation in her hands and feet. She has a reasonably good diet but doesn't have much time at the moment for exercise. She has no contraindications that restrict the treatment or require medical permission.

Reason for treatment: main aims of the treatment

My client requested a treatment that would help with fatigue. She also has dry skin and tense shoulders so she wants a treatment that will help with this also.

Rationale for the choice of each essence:

Rosemary-Invigorating, refreshing, Immune system, stimulates the mind, muscular aches.

Geranium- dry skin, stimulant, tonic, uplifting

Mandarin- uplifting, tonic, relaxing

Treatment plan:

One full body massage every week for 4 weeks. I will be massaging her legs, back, scalp, stomach, arms and face.

Oils / Botanical Name	Drops/ Mls	Uses
Rosemary / Rosmarinus officinalis	3 Drops	Stimulates the mind, congested skin, muscular aches, headaches, Immune system, Stress related disorders Invigorating refreshing
Mandarin / Citrus reticulata	2 Drops	Anxiety, insomnia, stomach ailments, uplifting, refreshing, stretch marks, Oedema, digestive
Geranium / Pelargonium graveolens	3 Drops	Circulation, lymphatic system, anti-inflammatory, pmt, menopause, nervous tension, stress related conditions.
Grape seed oil / Vitis vinifera	25 mls	Smooth oil, no odour, vitamin E, high in linoleic acid

I went through the safety factors with my client-
Rosemary is not suitable during pregnancy, on
epileptics or for someone with high blood pressure.
Mandarin is phototoxic so she needs to avoid strong
sunlight and sunbeds. Geranium is non-toxic, non-
irritating and non-sensitising so it is suitable to use. I
checked that these oils wouldn't affect her before I
started to use them.

TREATMENT 1

Details of how the therapist conducted the treatment

My client arrived for an evening appointment and I let her smell the blend of oils before I started. My client liked the smell of the blend so I proceeded to use it. The aim of the treatment is to help my client with mental fatigue so I choose Rosemary and Geranium specifically for this as both are stimulants and uplifting so they boost activity in the body and stimulate the mind.

Smell is the fastest way for essential oils to penetrate the body. The molecules in the oils send messages to the brain and from the lungs they pass to the bloodstream. Depending on the interpretation of the oil the brain will send messages to parts of the body to create a response. In this instance the responses to these oils would be clearing her mind, stimulating nerve endings and the brain, positive feelings and alertness, boosting her circulation. This was evident with my client at the end of the massage her expression was brighter, her mood had lifted, she was alert and felt she had more energy.

My client was very tense and had aches around the deltoid, trapezius and rhomboids on both sides when I worked over the muscles. I spent longer doing petrissage and frictions around these areas to cause erythema, drawing blood to the area to remove waste and bring more oxygen and nutrients in the blood to the tired stiff muscles. Rosemary is useful for muscular aches and pains as it has analgesic and antispasmodic properties which act as a painkiller and prevent /relieve spasms in tired muscles. The oil is also a rubefacient so it stimulates poor circulation which my client does have in her hands and her feet. This stimulating affect would boost blood flow around the body and create a feeling of warmth. The rest of the treatment went well and my client had no other tension.

How the client felt during the treatment

My client was very complimentary during the treatment and said she felt my pressure and technique was very relaxing. She was tense at her trapezius, rhomboids and deltoid muscles.

How the client felt after the treatment

After the treatment she felt her mood had lifted, she felt alert and not as tired as she had at the start of the massage. She said she felt she really needed the treatment as she hadn't much of a chance lately to relax and unwind.

Homecare advice

I advised my client not to shower or wash for the next 24 hours to fully absorb the oils. I gave her a sheet outlining general homecare advice and possible reactions to the treatment. Her skin is very dry and she tends to drink more coffee daily than water so I suggested she tries to drink a glass of water every time she has a cup of coffee to keep her hydrated. I suggested that when she is very tired during the day she should try to burn two drops of geranium or rosemary which I have used in the treatment to help lift her and keep her alert this would be more beneficial for her than drinking the amount of coffee she consumes to keep her alert. I suggested some light exercise like yoga to keep her supple and help with upper back tension.

I talked to my client about aspects that cause mental fatigue such as getting enough rest, eating a healthy diet, taking regular breaks and trying to reduce an excessive workload. She said she felt like this at the moment as she has a lot going on in college and work and she felt she wouldn't feel this way in a few weeks when she got on top of her workload.

Reflective practice

My client requested a treatment that would help with mental fatigue and I performed the massage in the evening using stimulating oils. I think next time it would be better to use stimulating oils in a morning or afternoon treatment instead of an evening treatment. I felt the bed was too low so I need to raise it up next time before I start a treatment. I had to break the routine to get some more oil as my clients skin absorbed it very quickly I need to keep contact with my client in future if I need to do this to avoid breaking the routine.

TREATMENT 2

Any changes to consultation

There are no changes to the consultation.

Reactions to last treatment

She was relaxed and alert she felt after the treatment. Also she felt the tension in her shoulders had eased afterwards which she wasn't expecting as she found the massage to be light and slow. I explained that I was using the oils to create the desired affect and I didn't need to do a deep massage to get the desired results. She said her mind wasn't as hazy for a few days after the treatment.

Details of the treatment

My client arrived for an afternoon appointment and she said she was happy for me to use the same blend of oils for this treatment. She said she was very tired today as she hadn't slept well over the last two nights this lead to her feeling more fatigued I still used rosemary and geranium for their stimulant properties to help with this and stimulate her mind.

I chose Mandarin for its uplifting and sedative properties and it eases all aspects of nervous exhaustion. She also said in the treatment she really liked the fruity smell, this positive association would help her relax and enjoy the massage more.

My client had very stiff calf muscles mainly her gastrocnemius muscles on both her legs she said she had started cycling this week and felt it was in relation to that. Rosemary is useful for muscular aches and pains as it is a rubefacient so it creates local warmth and boosts circulation in the area, this was evident as when I worked over the area with petrissage techniques there was erythema in the area, so the skin surface got redder as the blood circulated quicker bringing oxygen and nutrients to the muscles and removing waste.

My client was very tense and had aches around the deltoid, trapezius and rhomboids on both sides last week she had found this had eased and she wasn't as tense this week when I did Petrissage over the muscles. The rest of the treatment went well and my client had no other tension.

How the client felt during the treatment

During the Treatment she was very complimentary and said she was really enjoying the treatment and felt pampered. She had muscular tension in her gastrocnemius muscles on legs when I worked over them.

How the client felt after the treatment

She was in good spirits after the massage and said she felt very relaxed and less tense especially in her calf muscles. She felt she had a "boost" in the treatment and felt alert.

Homecare advice

I advised my client not to shower or wash for the next 24 hours to fully absorb the oils. My client had forgotten to increase her water intake this week and her skin was still dry she said she would try this week. I suggested that when she is very tired during the day she should try to burn two drops of geranium she had tried this twice this week and she didn't feel as mentally fatigued as usual. She didn't sleep well towards the end of this week so I suggested she mixes 6 drops of Mandarin with a un- perfumed shower gel and put it into a bath before bed. Mandarin is good for insomnia and it is uplifting so it can help with her sleep pattern.

Reflective practice

I used the same blend of oils last week but in an afternoon appointment which I feel was a better time for using stimulating oils. I made sure I had the bed at the right height this week so I didn't strain my back during the treatment.

I had broken contact with my client last week to get more oil but I remembered to keep contact this week which helped to keep the routine consistent. My client was very complimentary with the treatment throughout so I was very pleased with how the treatment went and I felt it boosted my confidence.

TREATMENT 3

Any changes to consultation

There are no changes to the consultation

Reactions to last treatment

Her calf muscles had been stiff last week but she felt that they were fine since the massage. She said she slept well the night of the last massage and for a few days since and her workload wasn't as heavy as usual so she didn't feel as fatigued as usual. She felt she had a positive mood after the last massage and she really liked it. Last night she hadn't slept very well. I did an evening appointment this week so I decided to change the blend slightly so as not to have a lot of stimulating oils in the evening.

The safety factors of these oils are Mandarin can be phototoxic so she needs to avoid strong sunlight or sunbeds. No known side effects with Lavender. Rosemary is not suitable during pregnancy, on epileptics or for someone with high blood pressure. I checked these with my client before I went ahead.

Oils / Botanical Name	Drops/ Mls	Uses
Rosemary / Rosmarinus officinalis	3 Drops	Stimulates the mind, congested skin, muscular aches, headaches, Immune system, Stress related disorders Invigorating refreshing
Mandarin / Citrus reticulata	2 Drops	Anxiety, insomnia, stomach ailments, uplifting, refreshing, stretch marks, Oedema, digestive
Lavender / Lavandula angustifolia	3 Drops	Antibacterial, germicidal, skincare, burns, wounds, stress, relaxation, insomnia, circulation, immune system, nervous system, refreshing and relaxing.
Grape seed oil / Vitis vinifera	25 mls	Smooth oil, no odour, vitamin E, high in linoleic acid

Details of the treatment

My client arrived for an evening appointment and she hadn't slept well the night before so I decided to change one of the oils to suit this. I also wanted to reduce the stimulating oils in the evening. I chose to change Geranium to Lavender in this treatment and keep the other oils the same. I explained that I wanted to use a more relaxing oil as it is an evening appointment and she was happy with the smell of the blend. I'm using Lavender oil to help her get to sleep and she said she always liked the smell; this association with the oil provokes a positive response so I chose it for this reason along with its properties that support the aims of the treatment. This oil balances the emotions and is good for sleep problems. Lavender elicits responses by influencing the brain and nervous system by changing the chemical messages sent around the body. In this case inhaling this oil has sedative and relaxing properties which help with sleep patterns. Lavender combined with Mandarin are depressants for the central nervous system- they decrease nerve impulses through the spine, brain and associated organs so as a result the person becomes more relaxed less nervous, making it easier to fall asleep and remain asleep.

My client didn't have any muscular tension in her upper back or her calves this week when I worked over the areas with effleurage and petrissage. She relaxed for the remainder of the treatment and I was able to perform a full body massage.

How the client felt during the treatment

She said she loved the smell of the blend and she chatted for a few minutes at the start of the massage asking benefits of the oils she then started to relax.

How the client felt after the treatment

After the massage she said she felt very calm and relaxed. Her breathing was much deeper and she seemed brighter and in better form. She said it was a great end to a very busy day.

Homecare advice

My client had increased her water intake this week and her skin didn't seem as dry as usual. I gave her the remainder of the blend of oils to use at home in an oil burner or to put the blend into her bath. She used geranium and rosemary this week in her oil burner and she felt quite alert afterwards and felt she wasn't drinking as much coffee to keep her alert. She started yoga this week and she felt it has helping to stretch out the muscles of her upper back.

I also suggested she made a hot compress and put two drops of rosemary on it and place it on her forehead and time she needs to clear her mind or feels stressed as it can help to relieve this.

Reflective practice

I was happy with how the treatment this evening went but I was a bit tired so I should really do treatment when I don't feel this way. My client was complimentary again for this treatment which helped boost my confidence and I feel more positive about my capabilities. My hands were a bit stiff so I need to do some stretches to keep them supple. I am more familiar with the oils so I was able to explain their benefits to my client without needing to refer to my book.

TREATMENT 4

Any changes to consultation

There are no changes to the initial consultation.

Reactions to last treatment

My client said she felt really relaxed and calm after the last massage she felt as a result of her mind being clearer she was able to sleep better that night. She said she hadn't felt fatigued since as she had got on top of her workload. She said she did feel a bit stressed later this week as she still has a lot of work to do in college. Her sleep pattern is much better but she requested a treatment this evening that was more for relaxation and also for stress. So I will be changing the blend to suit my client's needs. I checked the safety factors with my client -Cedarwood is avoid during pregnancy, Orange sweet can be phototoxic and Lavender has no known safety factors.

Oils / Botanical Name	Drops/ Mls	Uses
Cedarwood Atlas / Cedarwood Atlantica	3 Drops	Aches/pains/stiffness, anxiety, tension and stress, cystitis, urinary tract infections, Cellulite, oedema.
Orange Sweet / Citrus sinensis	3 Drops	Digestion, Nervous tension, Stress related conditions, refreshing, uplifting, sedative.
Lavender / Lavandula angustifolia	2 Drops	Antibacterial, germicidal, skincare, burns, wounds, stress, relaxation, insomnia, circulation, immune system, nervous system, refreshing and relaxing.
Grape seed oil / Vitis vinifera	25 mls	Smooth oil, no odour, vitamin E, high in linoleic acid

Details of the treatment

My client arrived for an evening treatment I changed the blend as she no longer felt fatigued and she was stressed this week. She also said she had tension and aches and pains in her back. I choose Cedarwood Atlas, Orange Sweet, and Lavender for this blend. My client smelled the blend and she was happy for me to use it. Orange Sweet has properties to help a client feel uplifted and is stress reducing. I chose Cedarwood Atlas for its Nervine and Sedative properties. Sedative properties of Cedarwood atlas along with the other oils blended would cause the brain to send out messages of relaxation, calm the nerves, causing deeper breathing and mind relaxing. This was evident with the client as the more she inhaled the oils she became calmer, breathed deeper and seemed to relax fully.

Lavender and Cedarwood atlas used in this treatment are good for reducing muscle pains and stiffness. The oil once absorbed into the bloodstream from the skin has a similar affect as the petrissage massage movements- the blood is warmed by the oil, it moves faster so oxygen /nutrients are brought to stiff muscles and waste in the muscles is removed faster. My client said she felt stiff in her lower back so I worked the latissimus dorsi and the external obliques with petrissage to ease the tension and improve the blood flow to the area. The rest of the treatment went well and my client had no other areas of tension.

How the client felt during the treatment

My client talked a good bit at the start of the massage and she moved a bit on the table after a few minutes she started to get comfortable and she stopped talking. She said she really liked the massage especially the frictions and petrissage techniques I used around her lower back.

How the client felt after the treatment

After the treatment she felt the tension in her lower back had improved and she felt in much better mood. She said she felt tired but in a relaxed way as she had a few busy day. She said she didn't feel as stressed as she had before the treatment.

Homecare advice

I advised my client once again to leave the oils on for 24 hours to get their full benefit. I had some oil left over from this treatment which I put into a bottle and asked her to use it over the next few days in an oil burner for relaxation and stress relief.

My client tried out the hot compress with rosemary on it and found it very beneficial for clearing her mind so she felt she would keep using it from time to time. My client is still going to yoga and has found it has been helping with upper back tension. My client requested this treatment for relaxation so I suggested she could use 6 drops of chamomile in her bath mixing it with an un-perfumed shower gel which would be great for relaxation and also help with sleep if she has any problems with that.

Reflective practice

My client was complimentary about the massage and I feel I really helped her relax. The room was a bit too hot so I needed to stop the routine to turn down the heating I need to check this in future before I start the massage so as not to break the routine. I spilled some of the oil on the floor during the treatment so I think it would be best to get bottle containers to pour the oil from when I start working instead of mixing the oil in a plastic bowl as the oil can often spill out.

OVERALL CONCLUSION

T1: My client requested a treatment to help with fatigue, dry skin and tense shoulders. I used rosemary, geranium and mandarin as they are useful for these aims. During the treatment she said she liked the pressure and techniques I used. She felt tense when I worked over her back and shoulders. After the treatment her mood had lifted and she was alert and not as tired. She felt she needed the treatment as she hadn't much of a chance to relax lately.

T2: She was relaxed and alert after the last treatment and the tension in her shoulders had eased. She felt her mind wasn't as hazy for a few days. She had tension in her calf muscles before and during the treatment. After the treatment she felt relaxed and less tense in her calf muscles.

T3: My client felt her stiffness had improved after the last treatment and she had slept well that night. She said she didn't feel as fatigued as usual. I changed the blend of oils to Rosemary, Mandarin and Lavender as it was an evening appointment and I didn't want her to feel too alert or stimulated after the treatment. She felt relaxed and calmer after the treatment. She had put rosemary and geranium into an oil burner the previous week which could contribute to her feeling less fatigued than usual.

T4: My client said she didn't feel fatigued after the last treatment and her mind had been clearer. She felt stressed towards the end of last week and she requested that she wanted the treatment for stress and relaxation as opposed to stimulating. I changed the blend to Cedarwood atlas, Orange sweet and Lavender. She had stiffness in her lower back and she found it hard to get comfortable at the start of the treatment. She felt she was in a better mood and she was relaxed and tired after the treatment but she didn't feel as stressed. I had suggested that she put Rosemary on a hot compress after the previous treatment and she had been using this and she felt it had helped to stimulate her and reduce her fatigue between treatments.

I noticed over the course of this Treatment that if the right oils are chosen and personal circumstances change the original aim of the treatment can change also. The original aim with this treatment was to help with reducing my client's fatigue, over the course of the four treatments she stopped feeling this way. It was a combination of her workload reducing, the massage with the specific oils and taking on some of my suggestions to use the oils at home. So by the last treatment my client requested a treatment that would be stress reducing and relaxing instead.

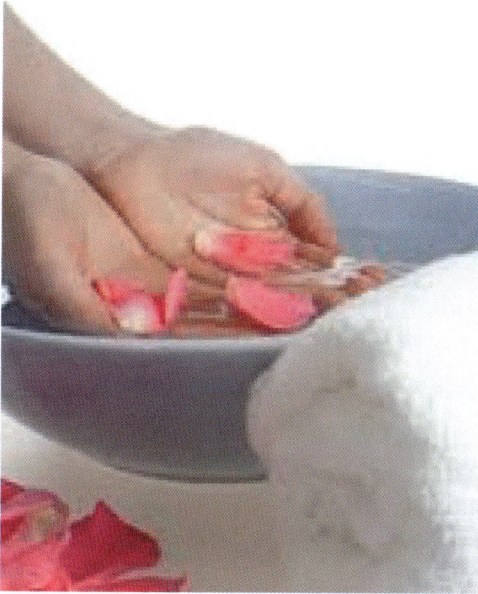

CASE STUDY 9

Client Profile

Annette O is a full time college student. She finds it hard to relax in general. She is currently doing two college courses so she feels she is under pressure with her workload. She rates her stress levels high between 7- 8. When she gets particularly stressed she gets eczema on her arms, hands and occasionally on her feet.

She regularly exercises doing spinning classes, walking, cycling. She eats three regular meals every day and doesn't smoke or drink caffeinated drinks. She has no contraindications that require medical permission or restrict the treatment

Reason for treatment: main aims of the treatment

My client has requested a treatment for relaxation, bring down her stress level and also she has sensitive skin prone to eczema so I needed to choose oils that would be suitable for this.

Rationale for the choice of each essence:

I have chosen Grape seed oil as the carrier oil it is a good quality oil that is odourless, colourless and quickly absorbed by the skin. It also contains some vitamin E which helps to protect and nourish the skin.

Chamomile Roman-calms skin conditions, stress, relaxing.

Sandalwood- Dry sensitive skin, stress.

Ylang Ylang- Stress reducing, mental relaxant, calming.

I did a patch test for Chamomile before starting this treatment as it can cause dermatitis, my client had no reaction to the oil so I proceeded to use it. Ylang Ylang can cause headaches and Nausea so I used only two drops in the treatment my client said she has inhaled this oil from a burner a few times and she hasn't had any adverse reactions to it. There are none known safety factors with Sandalwood.

Treatment plan:

One Aromatherapy massage once a week for four weeks. I will be doing a full body massage- Legs, Back, Stomach, Arms, Face, Neck and Scalp. 24 hours before I did the massage I tested the oils on my client with a patch test she had no reactions to the blend.

Oils / Botanical Name	Drops/ Mls	Uses
Chamomile Roman / Chamaemelum nobile	3 Drops	Allergies, Inflammations, Skin conditions, bruising, insomnia, stress, relaxing, sedative
Ylang Ylang / Cananga odorata	2 Drops	Euphoric effect, positive emotions, aphrodisiac, calming, relaxing
Sandalwood / Santalum album	3 Drops	Skin ailment, throat and chest infections, dry sensitive skin, Stress, depression.
Grape seed oil / Vitis vinifera	25 mls	Smooth oil, vitamin E, no odour, linoleic acid.

TREATMENT 1

Details of how the therapist conducted the treatment

I prepared the massage couch and helped my client onto the couch covering her with appropriate towelling. First I let my client smell the blend, she liked the smell, it had a mild smelling blend and got stronger as I applied it. I performed a full body massage checking the pressure of my movements and she said she preferred deeper pressure so I did this. Her gastrocnemius muscles on both legs were tense with a few adhesions on each so I worked the area for longer with petrissage and friction techniques. When I was doing frictions on her upper back she had some tension and stiffness around her scapulae bones. The main emphasis of the treatment is to reduce her stress level also choosing oils for her sensitive skin she finds the tension in her back is a result of feeling stressed and finding it hard to relax. She inhaled the blend I used Ylang Ylang as she said it is one of her favourite oils it is also useful for this blend as it has properties for creating positive emotions and it calms the central nervous system – the oil calms the nerve impulses through the spine, brain and associated organs so as a result the person becomes more relaxed and has less nervous tension.

She already likes this oil so if a client has a positive association with an oil they are more likely to relax and enjoy the treatment. Throughout the treatment with the combination of the oils and petrissage and effleurage techniques she seemed to calm right down and seemed to sink into the table breathing deeply in response to the treatment. When I had finished the massage I helped my client off the massage table and gave her a glass of water to drink.

How the client felt during the treatment

She said she really liked the massage and she felt very relaxed and calm. Her trapezius and sternocleidomastoid muscles were tense when I worked over them. She had eczema on her hands and was happy for me to apply the oils to her hands.

How the client felt after the treatment

She said she really enjoyed the massage and said she felt she needed it as she had been so stressed over the last few weeks and she hadn't had a massage in a long time. Her mood seemed to have lifted and she was in a better humour after the massage than what she had been beforehand.

Homecare advice

I gave my client a sheet outlining general homecare advice and possible reactions to the treatment. I asked her to leave the oils on for 24 hours to fully absorb them and get full benefit from their uses. She often burns essential oils at home and I suggested she tries Peppermint to clear and focus her mind while she is studying and Ylang Ylang for its relaxing sedative properties to help with her stress level. She spends at least 6 hours in front of the computer studying and I suggested that she tries to take regular breaks even take a lunch break where she goes for a walk to clear her head and also it will reduce any tension build up.

Reflective practice

My client was very complimentary about the treatment and said she liked the blend of the oils. She said after the treatment that she isn't normally keen on the smell of chamomile but she liked how it smelled with the other oils. Her response to the treatment I feel has boosted my confidence regarding doing aromatherapy treatments and blending oils. I was very relaxed while doing this treatment possibly due inhaling the blend along with the client. I am finding treatments easier to do as I am progressing through the course and I have more energy to do a few treatments in a row and I'm not as tense.

TREATMENT 2

Any changes to consultation

There are no changes to the consultation

Reactions to last treatment

She said she felt great after the last treatment she didn't feel as stressed for the rest of that day and slept well that night. She said she had tried a blend of Peppermint and Ylang Ylang in her burner between the treatments when she was studying and she found she was able to concentrate more on her work and wasn't getting as distracted.

Details of the treatment

My client arrived for an afternoon appointment she was in good spirits and said she was looking forward to the treatment. She had a positive response to the last blend of oils and was happy for me to use them again in this treatment. She said her eczema had cleared up slightly on her hands since last treatment. I choose oils specifically that wouldn't irritate and would improve the condition and also oils that would relax her as the condition flares up in response to her stress levels.

Chamomile Roman is effective for eczema as it helps clear up the skin condition on absorption and it also calms the person on an emotional level when it has been inhaled or absorbed through the skin. Chamomile has anti-inflammatory properties so it cools and sooths the skin. I also choose sandalwood for the same reason it is relaxing, sedative and it is beneficial for calming irritations in the nerves and skin such as eczema. When her stress level is low her skin condition clears up.

During the massage she had tenderness around the base of her scapulae the same location on each side and also she had some adhesions in the trapezius muscles at the base of her neck. I checked my pressure with my client and worked the adhesions and tenderness with deep frictions. She was tense all over her back but as I came to the end of the back massage her muscles were much looser and softer she felt the overall tension was due to her feeling stressed. The oils I've used have all got relaxing sedative properties, my client's brain picks up on the molecules of the oils when they are inhaled and sends messages through the nerves to create a response. The properties of these oils create a sense of calm and mental clarity on a physical level then it can encourage tense muscles to relax.

How the client felt during the treatment

She had some tension at her rhomboids and around her scapula bone and asked me to reduce my pressure while doing frictions over the muscles there. She was quite for most of the treatment but was a bit chatty towards the end of the treatment. She said while she was breathing deeply she started to notice than some areas of her body were very tense and other areas were very relaxed during the treatment.

How the client felt after the treatment

After the treatment she had some nasal congestion which started to develop while she was lying face down on the table. She appeared to be brighter and her face was flushed she said she felt alert and calm.

Homecare advice

She hadn't experienced any healing reactions after the last treatment and had a positive response to the blend of the oils.. She started to get nasal congestion during the treatment and she noticed this morning that her nose was blocked I suggested that she inhales Eucalyptus globulus as it is effective for catarrh and sinusitis. I explained to her not to use this oil on her skin as it can irritate sensitive skin but I suggested she can add two drops of the oil to a bowl of hot water and inhale the steam while covering her head with a towel so that the bowl is enclosed by the material.

She took two breaks while studying over the weekend and had burned the essential oils I suggested she said she felt a little less stressed than usual.

Reflective practice

I found the carpels in my wrist were clicking on my right hand when I was doing some of the massage movements and my hand felt stiff also so I think I will need to do a simple hand massage regularly and possible some stretches to keep my hands supple. My back got a bit tense during the massage but I am getting quicker at spotting when I feel like this and correct my posture and breathing deeply to relax. I applied too much oil when working around her neck and shoulders and my hands slipped a bit when I was trying to do the massage techniques.

TREATMENT 3

Any changes to consultation

There are no changes to the consultation.

Reactions to last treatment

She felt her stress level was lower for a few days after the treatment as a result her eczema wasn't as flared up as usual so she was much happier about this.

Details of the treatment

My client arrived for an afternoon appointment and was happy for me to continue using the same blend of oils as last time. I performed a full body massage leaving out the scalp at my client's request. I have chosen sandalwood the last few weeks for my blend due to its soothing properties for eczema and sensitive skin. It calms irritants such as nerves or skin irritations. Her skin has a tendency to be dry which can lead to it being sensitive. Skin like this is lacking in sebum which is a natural oil of the skin that helps create a natural moisture of the skin and acts as a protective barrier against bacteria and potential irritations. The chemical properties of Sandalwood sink into the skin and stimulate the sebaceous glands. This in turn increases the skins natural lubricant and making the skin healthier.

Reducing her stress levels also helps to reduce her eczema. Sandalwood has properties that are sedative and relaxing so it help reduce her stress levels. This combined with the similar properties of Ylang Ylang and Chamomile helps to calm her nervous system and on this occasion it relaxed her enough that she started to fall asleep.

My client was still tender at the base of her scapulae the same location on each side and also she had some adhesions in the trapezius muscles at the base of her neck. I checked my pressure with my client and worked the adhesions and tenderness with deep frictions and petrissage. The rest of the treatment went well and my client felt very relaxed at the end.

How the client felt during the treatment

During the treatment she fell asleep she said at the start of the massage she hadn't slept well the night before so that could have caused this. She was still drowsy when I turned her over on the table but said she felt great and really needed this time for relaxation.

How the client felt after the treatment

My client needed to go to the toilet straight away, when she returned I gave her a glass of water to drink and talked her through the homecare advice. She still was a bit tired but after she had the glass of water she started to become more alert. She said she felt very calm and she didn't feel as agitated as she had at the start of the massage.

Homecare advice

I suggested that if she finds it hard to sleep again she should try putting 2 drops of lavender or chamomile into her oil burner to help her sleep. I Had some oil left over from the massage so I suggested she used the oil up by putting it in her oil burner that day while she is studying to keep her stress levels low and help her concentrate more. She was working late last night trying to study and do her written work and she found this made it hard for her to sleep. I suggested that she tries to stop college work an hour before bedtime as working late is a mental stimulant. Also suggested if she is still very alert before bed having a relaxing bath and putting essential oils in will help her wind down.

The oils don't dissolve so I told her to mix 3 drops of Lavender and 3 drops of marjoram with an un-perfumed shower gel and add the mix to her bath as both can help relax her and help her sleep. My clients skin was drier this week than usual so I reminded her to try to drink 2 litres of water every day to keep her skin hydrated.

Reflective practice

I was better at judging the amount of oil this week so I didn't apply too much. I did some stretching exercises and hand massages on myself between the treatments so my hands didn't feel as stiff when I was doing the treatment. The treatment room got stuffy with the fan heater on so I need to make sure the room will be well ventilated next time. I got quite hot during the treatment and had to drink a lot of water after my client left – I need to stay hydrated myself this week. My client's skin absorbed the oil very quickly this week so I needed to make another 5mils for her face and neck. I need to make some more oil next time on the first blend if my client continues to have drier skin.

TREATMENT 4

Any changes to consultation

There are no changes to the consultation.

Reactions to last treatment

My client said she felt calm for the rest of the day and she felt she was better able to concentrate on her college work that day. She has continued to burn peppermint in her oil burner while she is studying or doing written college work and she has found she doesn't get distracted easily anymore and can get more work done as a result. She feels her stress level is high but she feels she might be like this till she gets all her written work done. She did feel however that after she has a massage she feels more relaxed for a few days afterwards. My client fell asleep during the last massage and she requested she wants to be more alert after the massage this time. So I will be changing the blend to suit my client's needs and still keep the original aims. I have chosen Geranium to replace Chamomile Roman. Chamomile is a sedative and a relaxant and I am changing it to Geranium which also helps stress and is suitable for sensitive skin without being a strong sedative.

Oils / Botanical Name	Drops/ Mls	Uses
Geranium / Pelargonium Graveolens	3 Drops	Circulation, lymphatic system, anti-inflammatory, pmt, menopause, nervous tension, stress related conditions.
Ylang Ylang / Cananga Odorata	2 Drops	Euphoric effect, positive emotions, aphrodisiac, calming, relaxing
Sandalwood / Santalum album	3 Drops	Skin ailment, throat and chest infections, dry sensitive skin, Stress, depression.
Grape seed oil / Vitis vinifera	25 mls	Smooth oil, vitamin E, no odour, linoleic acid.

Details of the treatment

My client arrived for an afternoon appointment I changed the blend slightly as my client didn't want to feel as tired as she did during the last massage. I was still conscious that I needed to use oils that were still suitable for eczema and sensitive skin. I did a patch test for this oil 24 hours before this treatment to make sure she didn't have a reaction to using the geranium oil. She didn't have a reaction so I proceeded. I let my client smell the blend and she said she was happy for me to use it.

Geranium like Sandalwood seeps into the skin and balances the sebum keeping the skin supple. This helps protect the skin and improve its condition. I choose Geranium also as I wanted oil that would help with her stress levels but not be a strong sedative. Geranium is a tonic for the nervous system it lifts the spirits and relieves anxiety and stress. She said her stress level was still high when she arrived but during the treatment her muscles started to relax more, her breathing got much deeper, she felt afterwards her mind was clearer and she felt her mood had lifted. After the oils are inhaled her brain would pick up on the chemical molecules and respond to the properties sending messages around her body through the central nervous system to create the desired response of relaxation.

My client had less tension in her shoulders this week when I worked over the area with petrissage and effleurage. She feels the tension gets particularly bad if she sits for a long time without taking breaks or doing exercise. She said that she has been trying to take regular breaks and doing stretches to help reduce this happening. Geranium has properties that are good for improving circulation improving circulation would help with bringing nutrients and oxygen in the blood to areas of tension and stiff muscles and help speed up removal of waste and toxins from tense muscles. For the remainder of the treatment my client was relaxed and she had no other areas of tension.

How the client felt during the treatment

She breathed deeply from the start of the massage and said she was really looking forward to the treatment. She said she really liked the back massage as she felt very tense today. When I went to turn her over on the table she said she really needed to go to the bathroom so I helped her up off the table and she went. She was very alert for the remainder of the treatment when she returned and she talked a bit.

How the client felt after the treatment

After the massage she said she felt great and less tense across her shoulders. She said she felt relaxed but alert also.

Homecare advice

My client took on board my advice for stopping college work an hour before bed and she has noticed she hasn't had any problems with her sleeping patterns since and she is able to relax more. She tried my suggestion for putting oil in her bath and she said she felt deeply relaxed after she tried it and plans to do this more in future. My client is taking regular breaks now while she is she is studying or working at her computer she finds she is more alert and works much better when she returns to it after a break. She is still using peppermint in her oil burner and is helping her feel focused. She said she still feels stressed but her mind is calmer so she is better able to keep up with the workload.

Reflective practice

There was some noise outside the room and I forgot some relaxing music so I need to play relaxing music next time and do the treatment in a room that won't have as much distractions outside in future. I was feeling tense before the treatment so I did some stretches for my shoulders and upper back beforehand. It really helped me relax and do a better treatment so I will try to do some stretching exercises in future before treatments.

OVERALL CONCLUSION

T1: The treatment aims were relaxation and reducing my clients stress levels. I needed to pick oils that were suitable for sensitive skin. I choose Chamomile, Sandalwood and Ylang Ylang. During the treatment she said she felt relaxed and calm she had tension in her Trapezius and Sternocleidomastoid. After the treatment her mood had lifted.

T2: My client slept well the night of the last treatment, and she was relaxed and didn't feel as stressed. She tried a blend of peppermint and ylang ylang between treatments when she was studying and she found she was able to concentrate more. She felt she had tension in her rhomboids and around her scapulae bones. After the treatment her face was brighter and flushed and she felt alert and calmer.

T3: After the last treatment she felt her stress levels were lower and her eczema wasn't as flared up as usual. During the treatment she fell asleep after the treatment she felt calm and alert.

T4: She said she was calmer than usual after the last massage and she was able to concentrate more on her college work as she had been putting peppermint into her oil burner between treatments. She was breathing deeply from the start of the massage , half way through the treatment she needed to go to the bathroom then she was alert for the remainder of the treatment and she felt less tense across her shoulders.

I was limited with the oils during the treatments as my client has sensitive skin but the oils I did choose seemed to reduce her stress levels every week and help with reducing her eczema breakouts. She was willing between treatments to take on board my homecare advice and this did help her between treatments to reduce her stress levels.

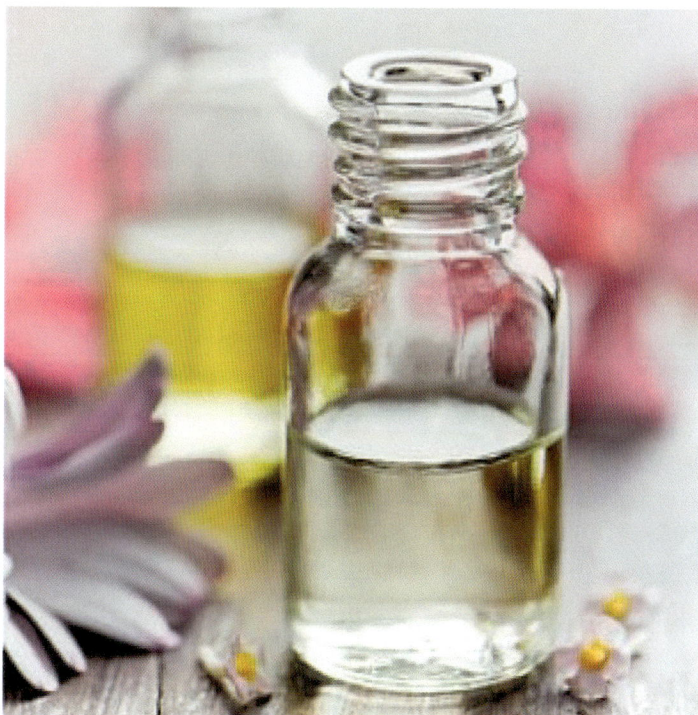

Case Study 10

Client Profile

May D is 60 years old. She has an active lifestyle going to the gym 3-4 times a week. She has a reasonably healthy diet and she doesn't drink or smoke. However she does drink a lot of tea and sugary foods. She is self-employed as a beauty therapist and makeup artist. She tends to work every day if clients request it and doesn't pass up work as some weeks she has very little and other weeks she has a lot of work.

Her husband died 2 years ago and she says she is still grieving and can be very upset and feeling depressed about this often. She occasionally feels stiff after her gym workouts but overall she doesn't have any noticeable aches and pains.

Reason for treatment: main aims of the treatment

My client suffers from grief and depression so my main aim is to help with this. She also experiences occasional stiffness so I will be trying to work on these issues when picking oils.

I checked the safety factors of the oils, Grapefruit and Rose Damask are non-toxic, non-sensitising, non-irritating and Chamomile can cause dermatitis in some people but she has used it on her skin before and hasn't had a reaction.

Rational for the choice of each essence:

Chamomile Roman - antidepressant, muscular aches and pains.

Grapefruit - uplifting, refreshing.

Rose Damask - antidepressant, relaxing, good for grief and sadness.

Carrier Oil Almond oil- this oil is easily absorbed by the skin, balances the moisture of the body and is suitable for all skin types

Treatment plan

One aromatherapy massage per week for four weeks; working on the legs, back, stomach, arms, face and head.

Oils / Botanical Name	Drops/ Mls	Uses
Chamomile Roman / Chamaemelum Nobile	2 Drops	Skin conditions, Bruising, insomnia, Stress, relaxing, antidepressant, muscular aches and pains.
Grapefruit / Citrus Paradisi	3Drops	Refreshing, uplifting, Nervous exhaustion, Depression, Oedema, Cellulite, Circulation.
Rose Damask / Rosa Damascena	3 Drops	Antidepressant, relaxing, good for grief and sadness, dry skin, mature skin, Pmt, menstruation.
Sweet Almond / Prunus Commmunis	25 mls	Protective, nourishing, vitamins- A,B1,B2, B6, E

Details of how the therapist conducted the treatment

My client arrived for an evening appointment, I prepared the massage table making sure I had enough towels and the room was warm. I aimed to perform a full body massage; before I started I washed my hands and sanitised my client's feet. I helped my client onto the massage table (protecting her modesty). I covered all body parts and only removed certain towels when I was massaging a particular area. I placed supports under her head, ankles and knees when needed. I let my client smell the blend before I started the massage and she liked it so I proceeded to use the oils.

The main aim of the treatment was to help my client with grief and depression. I chose Rose Damask for this. The oil has properties that are antidepressant and stimulate positive emotions thus helping to lift the client's mood and helping them feel better. My client's brain picks up on the molecules of the oils when they are inhaled and sends messages through the nerves to create a response. The properties of this oil help to lift a client's mood and calm the nervous system.

My client had no adhesions when I massaged over her muscles, she was tender when I massaged over her hamstring muscles but this was much looser after I worked the area with effleurage, petrissage and friction techniques. I chose chamomile for its antidepressant properties but it is also useful for muscular aches and pains as it is an analgesic so it will help to reduce them. The remained of the treatment went well and no other problem areas showed up.

How the client felt during the treatment

My client was very quiet from the start of the treatment she seemed very sad and tired at the start of the massage but she started to breathe deeply during the treatment and said she enjoyed it.

How the client felt after the treatment

Her expression was much brighter after the massage and she was definitely happier. She said she felt calm and relaxed and she felt her mood had lifted.

Homecare advice

I advised my client not to shower for 24 hours to absorb the full benefit of the oils. I gave her the remainder of the blend to put into an oil burner or into her bath at home to help lift her mood and help with depression.

My client appeared to be sad before the treatment so I advised her to put two drops of Rose damask onto a cotton ball on her radiator at home as means of inhaling the oil as it helps with grief and depression. I advised her to drink plenty of water for the rest of the day to help flush out accumulating toxins. My client has a healthy diet and exercises regularly which are positive ways for helping with her mental health but she said apart from meeting people through work she doesn't socialise often and keeps to herself so I suggested that maybe she could join a group that share an interest that she might have so she would have the opportunity to get out more and meet people.

Reflective Practice

I felt the treatment went well my client was more positive afterwards and seemed a lot happier and I was glad I was able to help her feel this way. I feel I picked oils that were best suited to her needs and I was confident in explaining their benefits to the client. As far as homecare advice is concerned I'm uncertain at this point on how much advice to give on dealing with depression and grief as I'm not qualified in dealing with these issues and I feel if my client needs some serious help with the matters I will refer her to a councilor or psychotherapist at a later stage.

TREATMENT 2

Any changes to the consultation

There are no changes to the initial consultation

Reactions to last treatment

My client said she felt much happier after the last treatment for the rest of that day and she put the oil I gave her into the bath the next night and she found it helped her to lift her mood for a few days. She felt her mood had dropped later in the week and she felt low again so she said she was looking forward to the treatment as she hoped it would help again.

Details of how the therapist conducted the treatment

My client arrived for the treatment and I felt it best to use the same oils again as she still had a low mood and she liked the smell of the oils I used last week. My client had muscular tension when I massaged over the bicep femoris, semitendinosus and semimembranosus. I needed to reduce my pressure when I did petrissage over the muscles, I did work the area for longer to draw more blood to the area. Warming the muscles helps the blood to flow quicker bringing more oxygen and nutrients to the area.

The analgesic properties of chamomile seeps from the dermis to the blood capillaries and this is transported to where it is needed and is a pain killer also the oil helps to bring down areas of inflammation.

My client can be depressed and suffers from grief, which is the main issue of the treatment. By inhaling the oils the properties reach the brain and the brain in turn illicit a response in the body. Rose damask is an anti-depressant so lifts the symptoms of depression such as low mood, negative thoughts, lack of concentration and feeling hopeless. I decided to combine this with Grapefruit as it has properties that are uplifting and refreshing which would help to invoke a positive attitude. It was evident that some change had come about during the treatment as she had gone from feeling very low when she arrived and looking very sad to have a brighter happier expression and she felt more calmer and relaxed.

How the client felt during the treatment

My client was quite from the start of the massage. During the treatment my client seemed a bit restless I asked her was she ok and she said she needed to go to the bathroom. So helped my client up and she went to the bathroom. When she returned I started the routine where I left off. She had tension in her hamstrings again which she felt was a result of working out a lot at the gym this week.

How the client felt after the treatment

After the treatment she was much more chatty than usual and she was much happier. She said she really enjoyed the treatment and felt it helped take her mind off things and she could relax fully during the treatment.

Homecare advice

I advised my client not to shower for 24 hours to get the full benefit of the oils and to drink plenty of water for the rest of the day to flush out toxins. She said she doesn't normally drink much water but I stressed the importance of doing this especially when she exercises a lot as she can get dehydrated very quickly. My client had said that her mood had lifted after the massage and had dropped later in the week. She explained that her mood can often vary. I gave her some suggestions that can help with depression. Firstly my client mainly eats very well but she eats a lot of sugary foods for snacks. The sugar gives a temporary boost to serotonin but the client can crash later so I advised her to cut down of try and stop eating refined sugars. I advised her to regularly record her moods and the triggers that cause her to feel that way, as she may begin to see patterns in what is causing her depression.

In addition, writing down her feelings can help her work through them. I advised her again to get some rose damask to put on her radiator at home to help lift her mood.

Reflective practice

I felt the treatment went well and she said she enjoyed the treatment. She was restless when I started the massage till I asked her if she was ok. She then said she needed to go to the bathroom, it seemed she was reluctant to say anything as I had already started but I explained this wasn't a problem and the treatment was her time and it would be best that she was comfortable that it wouldn't hindrance the treatment in any way. I looked up some information on depression between treatments to over her some simple helpful suggestions to help her. I just gave her two suggestions regarding this, as I didn't want to overload her with too much information at this point.

TREATMENT 3

Any changes to the consultation

There are no changes to the initial consultation

Reactions to last treatment

She felt the last treatment had really given her a boost and she felt more positive than usual. She did say that she felt very tired after the treatment last week which she said she didn't mind but she had a busy day ahead of her today and wanted to feel more alert after the treatment. She had tried out putting the Rose damask on her radiator a few times this week and she was delighted her mood had lifted when she used it. She said she felt tense this week when she arrived for the treatment as she had attended the gym a lot this week and felt she might have overdone the workouts.

I took my clients feedback into consideration and changed the oils but still kept in mind the original aim of helping with depression and grief.

I checked the safety factors- Eucalyptus smithii is not compatible with homeopathic treatments, which don't apply to my client, and orange sweet is phototoxic so my client needs to avoid strong sunlight or sunbeds.

Rational for the choice of each essence:

Eucalyptus smithii - stimulant, uplifting, analgesic helps relieve muscular aches and pains.

Orange Sweet - antidepressant, uplifting, sedative.

Rose Damask - antidepressant, relaxing, good for grief and sadness

Oils / Botanical Name	Drops/ Mls	Uses
Eucalyptus / Eucalyptus smithii	2 Drops	Headaches, head clearing, Immune system, muscular aches and pains, nervous system
Orange Sweet / Citrus Sinensis	3 Drops	Dull oily skin, digestion, nervous tension, stress related conditions, refreshing.
Rose Damask / Rosa Damascena	3 Drops	Antidepressant, relaxing, good for grief and sadness, dry skin, mature skin, Pmt, menstruation.
Sweet Almond / Prunus Commmunis	25 mls	Protective, nourishing, vitamins- A,B1,B2, B6, E

Details of how the therapist conducted the treatment

My client wanted to feel more alert after the treatment so changed some of the oils. I let my client smell the blend and she said she loved it and was happy for me to use it. I still kept Rose Damask in the treatment, as it is beneficial for helping with grief and depression. I also decided to use Orange sweet and Eucalyptus in the treatment. Orange and Eucalyptus are both uplifting oils so they would lift the client's mood and help the client have more positive emotions.

The Rubefacient property of Eucalyptus smithii brings warmth and redness to her skin as a result blood vessels dilate. More oxygen and nutrients are then brought to the area and removing waste which is especially beneficial for reducing muscular aches and pains in her biceps, triceps and hamstrings. I worked these areas for longer with extra petrissage movements to break down adhesions and manipulate and tone muscles. This combined with Eucalyptus produced erythema- increasing blood and lymph flow around her body.

My client had tension in her lower back in the external oblique's and Latissimus dorsi muscles, which she hadn't realised before the treatment. Eucalyptus smithii is an analgesic so the oil absorbs into the blood stream and has a pain killing effect on the muscles.

My client relaxed for the rest of the treatment and no other areas of tension were present.

How the client felt during the treatment

My client said she liked the pressure I used on her I used on her lower back and she hadn't realised she was tense there till I worked over the muscles. I needed to use less pressure on her arms and hamstrings this week as she felt they were stiff and achy. She seemed calm from the start of the massage and breathed deeply.

How the client felt after the treatment

She felt a lot less stiff after the treatment. She felt she was getting a tension headache coming on after the treatment, I explained that this sometimes can be a reaction to a treatment as it is caused by a release of toxins, apart from that she said she was happy with the massage and felt relaxed.

Homecare advice

My client has been feeling stiff after gym workouts so I suggested she could take a warm bath in the evenings to relax her muscles. I suggested she adds up to 6 drops of Lavender to an unscented shower gel to put into the bath. Lavender has relaxing, sedative properties and it helps with easing muscular aches and pains. I talked to her about the importance of warm up and cool down exercises before and after exercise, as this will help muscular tension.

I suggested last week that my client tries to cut down on refined sugary food she said she had noticed over the week that she often eats this type of food when she is feeling low and noticed it didn't do her any favours as she does crash afterwards and she feels sluggish afterwards so she has been trying to cut down. She wrote down how she has been feeling over the week and she has found it therapeutic. I suggested when she starts to feel depressed if she is at home to put two drops of grapefruit into an oil burner with 5mls of water to help lift her mood straight away this could counteract her sinking into depression for a number of days.

Reflective practice

I adapted the oils as my client felt too tired after the last treatment and she needed to feel her mood was lifted but more alert after this treatment. I was confident with explaining the benefits of the oils to my client. I was very thirsty during the treatment, which normally doesn't happen so I need to make sure I keep hydrated myself between treatments. I had the massage table lower than usual so I needed to bend my knees more to keep good balance and not strain my back.

TREATMENT 4

Any changes to the consultation

There are no changes to the initial consultation

Reactions to the last treatment

My client was happy that she felt positive after the last massage and very relaxed. She had a busy day ahead of her last week and she was glad that she still felt alert after the last treatment. She said she didn't feel as tense this week as she had taken my advice for putting a few drops of lavender into the bath a few times this week. She felt it help relax her muscles but also mentally she didn't feel as tense. She still puts Rose damask on her radiator and she said she plans to continue doing this as she loves the smell and feels it has helped lift her mood inhaling it.

Details of how the therapist conducted the treatment

I used the same blend of oils as last week as my client was happy for me to use them and she liked to the fact she was more alert after the last treatment. My client's mood has improved a lot as a result of the oils used and using them in between treatments. Rose damask has helped to evoke positive emotions in my client and counteract depression and grief.

My client had less muscular tension this week so I was able to apply more pressure when doing petrissage on her hamstring, biceps and triceps muscles. She said she felt the back massage was very relaxing this week and she started to fall asleep towards the end of it. Her lower back was tense again this week and the area was much colder there than the rest of her back which could suggest poor circulation. Eucalyptus smithii stimulates circulation. The warming effect of the oil helps the blood capillaries to dilate thus increasing the flow of the blood to the muscles.

How the client felt during the treatment

My client said she really enjoyed the treatment and the pressure I used on her legs this week was perfect and just what she needed. She seemed to relax fully during the treatment and nearly fell asleep while I was massaging her back.

How the client felt after the treatment

My client needed a few minutes to get off the massage table after the treatment and she said she felt very thirsty so I gave her two glasses of water to drink after this she started to feel more alert. She was happier after the treatment and said she felt much calmer and not as agitated as she felt before the treatment

Homecare advice

My client said she had made a lot of effort this week to try and cut down on sugary foods and she said she felt much better as a result. She has tried out using Grapefruit in an oil burner and rose damask on her heater and she has felt they have helped between treatments to lift her mood. I also suggested this week that talking about the way she feels to a friend or family member she could trust can help also to lift her mood and sort out some issues she has. She said that she hasn't done this much lately and doesn't want to burden anyone with how she feels. This could leave her feeling isolated and lonely and I said she might be surprised if she starts talking to people as I feel they would be more understanding and helpful than she thinks. She said she would take this on board and give it a go. Her muscular tension has improved as she is doing more stretches after her workouts and took my advice for putting Lavender in her bath. I gave her the remainder of the oil from the treatment to put in her oil burner over the next few days.

Reflective practice

I was happy with how this last treatment went. I felt I had muscular tension in my back before I started the treatment so I spent ten minutes doing stretches before I started to help relax my muscles and reduce the tension. I felt I did a much better treatment as a result. I made sure to have the table higher up this week and I felt this helped my posture. My client has taken on board my advice for using the oils over the last few weeks and I am glad she has had a positive response to them and they have helped her a lot.

CONCLUSION

T1: The aims of the treatment were to help with grief, depression, and occasional stiffness. I chose Rose Damask, grapefruit and chamomile Roman. At the start of the massage she was tired and sad. After the treatment her expression was brighter and she was calmer and relaxed. Her mood had lifted.

T2: After the last massage she was happier and her mood had lifted. She used the blend of oils I gave her in the bath. Later in the week she had a low mood again. Start of the treatment she was quiet and restless and she had tension in her hamstrings. After the treatment she was chatty and happier.

T3: She felt positive after the last treatment but she felt tired also. She requested a treatment that would keep her more alert as she had a busy day ahead of her so I changed the blend to Eucalyptus smithii, Orange sweet and Rose damask. She had aches and pains in her arms, thighs and lower back. She felt less tense after the treatment and was happy and relaxed. She felt she was getting a tension headache after the massage.

T4: She felt happy, positive and relaxed after the last treatment and had put lavender into her bath to help with muscular aches and pains. During this treatment she relaxed and nearly fell asleep. After the treatment she felt alert, happy and calmer. My client has had a positive response to the oils over the four treatments and her mood seems lifted after each treatment she was also willing to take on some of my suggestions to help her during the week to lift her mood.

FREE BONUS: CONSULTATION FORMS

Download link to your free files: CLICK HERE

FINAL WORDS

Can I Ask A Favour?

If you enjoyed this book, found it useful or otherwise then I'd really appreciate it if you would post a short review on Amazon. I do read all the reviews personally so that I can continually write what people are wanting.

Thanks for your support!

Printed in Great Britain
by Amazon